Nature's Alternatives
to Phen-Fen

RITA ELKINS, M.H.

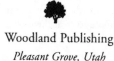

Pleasant Grove, Utah

Contents

INTRODUCTION

It has been less than a year since I published my first booklet on phen-fen. In it, I strongly suggested that anyone who was taking the drug should seriously reconsider. Shortly before the publication of this book, and in the wake of frightening clinical data, the FDA removed phen-fen from the market. The alarmingly high incidence of valvular heart damage and pulmonary hypertension linked to phen-fen usage prompted this dramatic withdrawal. Unfortunately, scores of people—confident the FDA had done its job—had already taken the drug for various lengths of time. For many of these people, the physiological damage sustained by their bodies may be irreversible.

In 1996, the total number of prescriptions for phen-fen written in this country exceeded 18 million. Statistics suggest that as many as 30 percent of patients using phen-fen may have lesions on their heart valves caused by combining fenfluramine and phentermine. People who thought they had finally found the ultimate weight loss panacea find themselves back at square one again. So the question arises once more: "Are there any safe substances that can effectively inhibit appetite, supply energy, and boost caloric burning without compromising health?" The answer to that query is a definitive "YES."

What this book endeavors to do is cover virtually every natural substance which can help to facilitate safe weight loss. It covers natural appetite suppressants, fat burners, fat absorbers, blood sugar regulators, muscle builders and substances which promote good elimination. My hope is to provide an informative survey of natural weight loss supplements so that you, the consumer, can decide what you want to try, know it when you see it, and understand its mechanics. Choosing to lose weight wisely is what its all about. Becoming weight conscious should be synonymous with becoming health conscious.

Chapter 1

The Phen-Fen Fiasco

Everyone seemed to be clamoring for the chemical compound called phen-fen, hailed as the most revolutionary diet pill to emerge in several decades. Prescribing dexfenfluramine became so common that safety concerns were exchanged for possible quick and dramatic weight loss. The real consequences of the reckless application of this powerful drug are just now emerging. The casual use of dexfenfluramine and fenfluramine (also known as Redux and Pondimin) had many health-minded individuals alarmed, and the concern was justified.

While pharmacologists strongly advised that no one should take a drug that alters brain chemistry unless they absolutely need it, everyone was hopping on the phen-fen bandwagon. Dexfenflu-ramine was shamefully easy to get. Its purported ability to melt away pounds made it the most popular pill in America. What was overlooked is that phen-fen was originally intended for patients that qualify as being truly obese. It was not manufactured for those who want to lose twenty pounds or less. Some responsible doctors believe that phen-fen is the most over-prescribed drug to date, due to a profound medical negligence linked to its indiscriminate dispersion. Another problem is that proper nutrition and exercise should accompany any weight loss supplement. Current trends, however, show that many people used phen-fen as a way to lose weight with little or no attention given to sound nutrition or exercise.

No studies exist which evaluate the safety of using phen-fen over extended periods of time. Like other drugs which quickly emerge, touted by pharmaceutical companies, and go on to experience tremendous consumption, phen-fen was once considered a safe compound. In light of recent events, the question of how the drug was allowed to become so prevalent must be addressed.

WHAT MAKES PHEN-FEN SO DANGEROUS?

What is commonly known as phen-fen is actally the drug dexfenfluramine—a combination of the two chemicals phentermine and fenfluramine. During the 1960s, the FDA approved each of these drugs as separate therapeutic agents to be used individually. Originally, these drugs were used to treat psychological disorders such as obsessive-compulsive behavior and even cocaine addition.

This mixture of phentermine and fenfluramine works to adjust the levels of two very vital neurotransmitters in the brain: serotonin and dopamine. In 1992, Dr. Michael Weintraub combined these medications to create a drug he felt would be effective for long-term weight loss. The fenfluramine component of the mix helps to raise serotonin levels, creating a feeling of fullness, while the phentermine acts on dopamine and norepinephrine somewhat like an amphetamine stimulant. Some experts believe that the "phen" part of this combo was added to help the fatigue that fenfluramine can cause. This particular drug duo regulates and attempts to balance out the serotonin and dopamine present in the body. Creating the proper balance between these neurotransmitters is critical to both physical and emotional health.

As far as safety goes, neither dexfenfluramine nor fenfluramine is a completely safe compound. To the contrary, long term studies on the health risks of using these drugs in combination is seriously lacking. Several pharmacologists cautioned the American public that further testing of this drug was warranted in order to determine whether phen-fen could lead to problems such as derangements in brain chemistry, adverse effects on memory, inhibition of sexual function, initiation of depression or behavioral changes, and serious damage of the cardiac and pulmonary systems.

English medical practitioners were allowing a maximum of only three months on this drug, compared with American doctors who set no time limits on phen-fen therapy. While the FDA gave dexfenfluramine its seal of approval, most people who did take the drug for extended periods of time put up with a number of negative side effects. Diarrhea, dry mouth, drowsiness, fatigue and personality changes were common. Many doctors simply advised that these symptoms would ease with time.

Today we are a wiser group of consumers who realize that the potential hazards of a pharmaceutical agent designed to reorchestrate brain chemistry should not have been taken lightly. Moreover, it was dangerous of us to assume that just because the two drugs were considered safe when taken individually, we could ignore the potential hazards of combining them into one compound. Long-term testing on the effects of taking these compounds together was conspicuously lacking and the consequences of this blatant lack of clinical documentation should have been more sobering.

One potentially life-threatening side effect of phen-fen is primary pulmonary hypertension. Lesions which develop on the heart valves are of even more concern. Combining phen-fen with other drugs may also create other serious side effects. Even before the FDA took phen-fen off the market, the health hazards of taking dexfenfluramine with melatonin were under research at the University of Utah in Salt Lake City. People suffering from depression or high blood pressure were cautioned against taking phen-fen. Other side effects linked to phen-fen include: nerve damage, severe cramping, fever, vomiting, a "spaced out" feeling, and temper outbursts.

Anyone who is currently taking the drug must now slowly taper off and this can result in extreme exhaustion, insomnia, irritability and personality changes. (*Note:* While current combinations of phen-fen have been taken off the market, new combinations are in the works. The watchword here is *extreme caution.* Even if a new chemical mix emerges which is purported as safe, mixing any other drug with fenfluramine will inevitably come with significant risks.)

How Phen-Fen Works

Rather than working on the stomach, phen-fen works on the brain by suppressing a specific brain signal that triggers hunger sensations. In other words, by manipulating brain cell chemistry, phen-fen inhibits our impulse to eat. It does this by keeping serotonin levels up and continually recirculating serotonin supplies. Serotonin that would normally be lost from brain tissue remains and its effects last longer. This abnormal serotonin glut is what shuts down the sequence of events which result in overeating or continual snacking. There is a loss of interest in eating and a dramatic decline in caloric intake, so pounds are shed. The problem is that this type of weight loss comes with a big price tag. How much of our health are we willing to compromise in order to be slim and trim? If we become well-informed and use our heads, we will not only lose weight safely, but will actually enhance our health at the same time.

Safe and Effective Alternatives to Phen-Fen

This book is for those individuals who prefer to forgo powerful pharmaceutical agents in exchange for natural compounds that accomplish physiological results similar to those of phen-fen. These natural options can be effective and are certainly preferable to potent, synthetic chemical compounds. This book offers the reader a survey of natural supplements that work to accomplish the same aims as phen-fen and other new diet drugs like orlistat, leptin and sibutramine. While no one questions the serious health risks associated with obesity, certain questions must be addressed before we engage in any weight-loss plan based on powerful drugs or other drastic measures.

- Is it wise to expose your body and its systems to long term drug therapy without knowing the hazards of prolonged use?
- Does the amount of weight you need to lose justify the use of a powerful drug?
- Are you willing to become dependent on pharmaceutical agents for the rest of your life in order to.maintain an ideal weight?
- Have you investigated other safer natural compounds that can suppress food cravings and overeating?
- Could you apply the $30 to $100 a month it costs to take diet drugs to other safe, nutritional supplements that can effectively curb your appetite?

It is also important to consider the following points:

- A weight reduction program should not compromise physical health for weight loss.
- Most fad diets and diet drugs are unnatural and provoke a host of undesirable physical responses.
- Sound weight loss should work with, not against, body systems and life style. Weight loss strategies should act in partnership with the body, not debilitate it.

Chapter 2

Suppressing the Appetite Naturally

I was long under the misconception that it is our stomachs that dictate whether we feel hungry or not. To the contrary, food cravings and appetites are intrinsically linked to neurochemical changes in the brain which stimulate our appestats and subtly (or not so subtly) prompt us to eat.

Most of us frequently crave much more food than we actually need to sustain life. This results in excess calorie consumption and subsequent fat storage. Scientists now believe than when we experience a desire to eat that is not based on our body's actual need for fuel, we may be experiencing a brain chemistry phenomenon. In other words, many of us feel prompted to eat as an after-effect of stress, mental fatigue, depression, PMS, etc. What we really need isn't food at all, but rather a raise in serotonin levels.

Anytime serotonin levels in brain tissue dip significantly, certain events occur. We can feel depressed, fatigued, grumpy, jittery, etc. Eating certain foods like carbohydrates can help to raise brain serotonin, resulting in a restored feeling of well-being. Some of us are much more sensitive to serotonin drops than others. The desire that drives us to rummage for stale chocolate, binge on a bag of cookies, and stuff ourselves with potato chips may be based on our very real need to adequately raise serotonin. The idea of "comfort foods" may be just that—foods which are able to make us feel better, sleep better and even cope better. In the past, this type of eating was called "emotional consumption" and was relegated to a form of psychological dependence. Today, we know that this behavior is stimulated by a complex series of biochemical events.

Of particular relevance is the fact that when we become overweight, we may be inadvertently promoting carbohydrate consumption through faulty brain chemistry. Interestingly, animals allowed to choose between carbohydrate and protein-rich foods instinctively regulate not only their calorie consumption but also the proper ratio between protein and carbohydrates. In contrast, overweight individuals frequently consume half or more of a day's intake of food in the form of carbohydrate-rich foods and snacks, almost always as a result of a strong craving.

More and more research points to the notion that this abnormal desire to overeat carbohydrate foods may be related to a brain abnormality which interferes in the normal process of serotonin release. Apparently, many of us may be suffering from drops in serotonin levels which prompt us to keep raiding the cookie jar. Hormonal factors, personality and heredity all play a role in determining when, what and why we eat.

Drugs like phen-fen are developed in an attempt to artificially regulate the brain chemicals linked to sensations of hunger. But as is the case with most synthetic pharmaceutical drugs, phen-fen initiates a whole series of physiological reactions in the body— many of which are undesirable. For this reason natural supplements which work to suppress the appetite and curb food cravings are a much better choice. These supplements *naturally* suppress the desire to eat and stimulate the burning of fat. When compared to potent drugs like phen-fen, they are infinitely safer.

The next few sections of this booklet will address several categories of weight control and how they can be managed through natural means. We'll look at specific compounds which raise serotonin levels, suppress the appetite, absorb fats after ingestion, enhance the metabolic furnace, and boost digestion and elimination. Be assured that effective and safe natural compounds do exist which can significantly contribute to weight loss and maintenance.

AMINO ACID THERAPY

Amino acid therapy works by creating an excess of amino acids, which, in turn, forces the body to create increased amounts of brain chemicals like serotonin. Drugs like phen-fen are designed to do much the same thing; however, they are much more potent and invasive in their cellular effect. Because of their synthetic chemical structures, they initiate a whole host of physiological reactions, many of which are not desirable. Taking certain amino acids can also alter brain chemistry but the mechanisms by which this is accomplished work with the body rather than against it.

Numerous studies have found that there are several ways in which amino acids can be used to help control hunger and appetite surges. Certain amino-acid supplements act as precursors to the very neurotransmitters affected by phen-fen. Brain amines like serotonin are ultimately produced from amino acids which, ideally, come from the protein components of our diet. The production of certain brain amines can also be stimulated through proper supplementation of specific amino acids. It is vital to understand that if amino acid therapy is to be effective, certain vitamins and minerals must be provided. Remember, serotonin levels are the key to the stimulation of appetite and feelings of well-being and satisfaction. Since serotonin, dopamine and norepinephrine are the specific brain amines involved in appetite control, elevating their precursors through dietary supplementation is essential.

Tyrosine and Phenylalanine

Recent research conducted at MIT concludes that tyrosine plays a profound role in determining the rate at which four crucial brain chemicals are produced. It directly affects the blood levels of these neurotransmitter compounds, especially serotonin. This amino acid also boosts glandular production of adrenaline which can cause a rise in dopamine levels. Some doctors have success-fully used tyrosine to treat depression, a condition intrinsically linked to serotonin levels.

Phenylalanine, like tryptophan and tyrosine, also acts as a precursor to brain amines. Phenylalanine can actually convert to tyrosine and contribute to the formation of 2-PEA, a compound believed to be a neurotransmitter closely related to norepineph-rine. It is worth noting that chocolate cravings may be related to phenylalanine deficiencies. Anecdotal studies have suggested that women who suffer from PMS, depression, consistent food cravings and weight gain may also be chronic "chocoholics." Chocolate contains high concentrations of PEA or phenylalanine, the amphetamine-like stimulant properties of which boost energy levels and elevate mood.

The traditional association between chocolate and romance may be based on the feeling of well-being that phenylalanine creates. If you find yourself ransacking your night table drawers for a bit of chocolate, or mixing up cocoa and sugar as a mid-afternoon snack, you may be low in phenylalanine. More impor-tantly, if you are low in either phenylalanine or tyrosine, you may be susceptible to depression or carbohydrate cravings.

Guidelines: Take 500 to 1000 mg of phenylalanine thirty min-utes before a meal to reduce hunger or take 500 to 3000 mg of tyrosine before breakfast and lunch.

Safety Issues: Tyrosine should not be used by anyone taking beta-blocker drugs, or who is suffering from hypertension. Neither should phenylalanine be taken by anyone with high blood pressure, diabetes, or PKU. Pregnant or nursing mothers or anyone suffering from melanoma should also avoid these amino acids.

Methionine

Methionine has also been linked to weight control. More than one study using phenylalanine and methionine has found that a significant reduction in food intake resulted for overweight individuals using both amino acids.[1] The physiological mechanism responsible for this effect is thought to be the stimulation of a gastrointestinal hormone called cholecystokinin which may actually cause the brain to stop the desire to continue eating. Clinical studies support this idea and also show that methionine assists in the breakdown of fats.

L-Arginine, L-Ornithine and L-Lysine

All three of these amino acids should be taken together since the trio helps to burn fat stores. Arginine assists in weight loss by boosting the creation of muscle mass while reducing fat stores. Ornithine helps promote the release of growth hormone which helps the body burn excess fat. Lysine contributes to the creation of muscle protein and helps to lower high serum triglyceride levels.

Safety Issues: Anyone suffering from viral infections (especially herpes) or who is pregnant or nursing should not take arginine. Ornithine is not for children, pregnant or nursing mothers, or anyone with a history of schizophrenia.

How to Use Amino Acids

Amino acids work best if they are taken with a little fruit juice and nothing else. Never take amino acids with a protein food, or their effectiveness will be compromised by competing amino acids. Tyrosine is considered somewhat milder than phenylalanine as far as possible side effects. People suffering from high blood pressure or anyone taking MAO antidepressant drugs should not take these amino acids without their doctor's supervision. Free-form amino acids do not have to undergo complex digestive processes for assimilation as they are already designed for immediate use. Supplementing tyrosine and phenylalanine with vitamin B6 and B12 is also recommended to enhance effectiveness.

HERBS AND THE APPETITE

Several herbs are considered appetite inhibitors and can be added to a weight loss program. Frequently, weight loss formulas or natural appetite suppressants will add one or a combination of these herbs in order to discourage food cravings. The following list includes the more common hunger-controlling herbs:

CHICKWEED: Used as a natural appetite suppressant.

PLANTAIN: Studies have found that using plantain resulted in greater weight loss due to satisfying hunger and reducing the absorption of fats.[2] It is considered a natural appetite satiator.

ASTRAGALUS: Helps to increase energy and stamina and promotes better nutrient absorption which can prevent necessary food cravings.

FENNEL: Removes mucus and fat from the intestinal tract and also acts as a natural appetite suppressant.

The amino acids and herbs listed in this chapter are considered good appetite suppressants; however, many of the other supplements discussed under other headings also work to curb our desire to eat. Tyrosine and phenylalanine work in ways similar to phen-fen but are much safer. We now know that controlling serotonin has a profound impact on the desire to eat, especially when it comes to carbohydrate cravings. If you consider yourself an emotional or mental eater, you may want to try amino acid therapy combined with one or a combination of the herbs listed. Remember that before we can effectively lose weight, we must understand why we crave and eat certain foods.

Chapter 3

Dietary Fat: A Health Enemy

Virtually all health experts agree that a high-fat diet is directly linked to cardiovascular disease, various types of cancer and premature death. The National Institute of Health, the World Health Organization and other scientific institutes have confirmed the frightening hazards of fat. Obesity and cardiovascular disease, two of the most insidious killers of Americans, can be linked to Western eating habits and the overconsumption of fatty, salty, and sugary foods. Thousands of Americans are dying before their time or living extremely compromised lives just because they ingest too much fat and exercise too little. Greasy, fried, rich foods have burdened our bodies with excess fat that clogs arteries and causes hypertension, heart attacks, strokes and cancer. Looking at the phenomenal amounts of money spent on weight loss programs, the notion that we consume too much fat is becoming redundant, to say the least. Still, many of us remain oblivious to the fat grams we routinely pop into our mouths.

TOTAL FAT GRAMS IN SINGLE SERVINGS

Bacon Cheeseburger/Hardees	39
Burrito Supreme/Taco Bell	22
Hamburger Deluxe/Wendys	21
Quarter Pounder with Cheese/McDonalds	28
Sausage Biscuit with Egg/McDonalds	33
Popcorn Chicken/KFC	45
Whopper/Burger King	36

Source: Center for Science in the Public Interest and *McDonald's Nutrition and You—A Guide to Healthy Eating at McDonalds*, 1991, McDonalds Corp.

To make matters worse, many of us were raised on seemingly innocuous foods that are loaded with fat. Some of these include:

- battered fish sticks
- ramen soup
- pepperoni pizza
- pancakes, waffles and muffins
- pies and pastries
- candy bars (60 percent of the calories come from fat)
- hot dogs
- cheesy casseroles
- burritos
- doughnuts
- ice cream
- macaroni and cheese

Fat is the major ingredient in most of the snack food we constantly nibble on. Check ingredient labels to find the fat gram content of most snack foods—you'll be surprised to find out how fatty they are. Even a healthy sounding food like a bran muffin can contain thirty-six grams of fat! No wonder they stay so moist. Fat adds wonderful flavor to food and is often liberally used in the form of butter, sour cream, whipping cream, melted cheese, cream cheese spreads, dips, cream sauces and gravies. Did you know that only one-half of an avocado has fifteen grams of fat? And one measly glazed doughnut has thirteen grams of fat.

Research continues to point to fat as a more dangerous culprit than anyone might have imagined. Saturated fats such as lard, beef tallow, and palm and coconut oils are particularly menacing. Researchers have found again and again that fats can contribute to the growth of tumors in animal studies.[3] A recent article in the *New England Journal of Medicine* reports that even a relatively small amount of extra body fat increases the risk of certain diseases for women and may compromise longevity. Even being mildly overweight may be much more risky than anyone previously assumed.[4]

FAT-RELATED DISEASES

Ideally, only 20 percent or less of our total caloric intake should come from fats. Eating too much fat can cause:

- obesity
- heart disease
- hypertension
- decreased longevity
- formation of free radicals
- colorectal cancer
- cervical cancer
- prostate cancer
- gallbladder disease
- coronary artery disease
- stroke
- joint inflammation (arthritis)
- breast cancer
- ovarian cancer
- endometrial cancer

Fats and Arthritis

Most of us aren't aware that dietary fats contain certain components which serve to create substances in the body called prostaglandins and leukotrienes, which are involved in the process of inflammation. The joint pain associated with rheumatoid arthritis is created by these hormone-like compounds. Therefore, eating a high-fat diet can contribute to the body's inflammatory responses.

Breast Cancer, Dietary Fats, Fiber and Indoles

Dr. Leonard Cohen of the Nutritional Endocrinology Department at Naylor, Dana Institute of the American Health

Foundation, believes that precancerous lesions found in breast tissue will develop into cancer only if they are stimulated by certain agents such as fat.[5] Women increase their risk of developing breast cancer when they consume a diet high in fat and animal protein, but low in fiber, vegetables and fruits.

> According to a landmark study that investigated the link between breast cancer and dietary fat in 8900 nurses, a reduction in fat intake from 40 percent to 30 percent of total calories is not sufficient to lower risk. It is likely that fat intake must be below 25 percent of total calories before breast cancer risk is reduced. This requires considerable changes in the typical American diet.[6]

In addition, estrogen plays a key role in breast cancer. When women put on weight, they have a tendency to create more estrogen, and certain forms of estrogen can act as carcinogens. The type of estrogen commonly found in overweight women, or in those who eat a high-fat, high-protein diet, can initiate changes in breast tissue which can lead to the formation of cancerous tumors. The three most important ways to inhibit "bad" estrogen from inducing breast cancer are:

1. Maintain an ideal body weight.
2. Eat a diet high in fiber and low in fat. Fiber helps to sweep excess estrogen from the bowel so it does not recycle.
3. Consume enough cruciferous vegetables (broccoli, cabbage, cauliflower, brussels sprouts, kale, radishes, watercress, etc.) so that adequate amounts of indole-3-carbinol enter the system.

Colorectal Cancer and Fat

Dietary fat intake has been closely related to the incidence of colon cancer. When we ingest fat, especially animal or saturated fat, cholesterol and bile acid production is accelerated in the liver. Consequently, as food is processed these substances are stored in the bowel. Due to the action of intestinal flora, these compounds can be chemically altered to form carcinogenic chemicals which damage the lining of the colon and promote the formation of cell mutations.

Cervical, Uterine, Endometrial, Prostate Cancers

As mentioned earlier, the heavier a woman is, the higher her levels of a harmful type of estrogen will be. This estrogen plays a role in the development of endometrial, cervical and uterine cancers. It has been reported by the National Academy of Science that "diet is responsible for 60 percent or more of all cancer in women. The most important dietary change you can make to protect against these diseases is to reduce dietary fat to less that 30 percent of total calories, preferably to less than 25 percent."[7]

The incidence of prostate cancer has also been linked to fat consumption and is intrinsically connected to free radical formation, cholesterol metabolites and hormonal factors in males.

Cardiovascular Disease and Fat Consumption

The National Institute of Health (NIH) has stated that almost all of the top ten causes of death due to disease are attributable to health risks linked to excess body fat. In other words, if we let ourselves become obese, we are much more prone to developing heart disease, high blood pressure, stroke, diabetes and various forms of cancer. Cardiovascular disease is the leading cause of death and disease in out country. 512,000 people die of heart attacks every year. Our blood cholesterol levels are the primary indicators of our risk of cardiovascular disease. And to make matters worse, the more fat we eat, the higher our cholesterol rises and the more free radicals we create. Free radicals damage our artery walls and compound the problem of cardiovascular disease.

Diabetes and Body Fat

Being overweight is one significant contributor to the development of adult-onset diabetes. In some individuals, carrying excess body fat inhibits the ability of cells to take sugar from the blood, even if adequate amounts of insulin are present. Many individuals with this type of diabetes are cured just by losing weight. Simply put, being overweight significantly increases our risk of developing diabetes and several other degenerative diseases. As we get older, some of us tend to collect more body fat above the waist. This type of fat accumulation is associated with diseases like diabetes, heart disease, gallbladder disease and some kinds of cancer.

Gallbladder Disease and Fat Consumption

Every time fats are consumed, cholesterol levels increase in bile stores. Gallstones are formed from bile acids which can form into stones when cholesterol is present. Eating a diet that contains too many fatty foods can tax both the liver and gallbladder and cause stones to form. Lowering fat consumption and boosting fiber intake can help to prevent gallbladder disease.

Cholesterol: HDL and LDL Varieties

Cholesterol is not technically found in food, but is produced by the body. However, the types of fats we eat influence how much and what type of cholesterol our bodies make. Saturated fats are particularly good at raising a variety of cholesterol called low-density lipoprotein, or LDL cholesterol. The more of this type of cholesterol we have floating around in our bloodstream, the greater our risk of developing atherosclerosis, heart attack and stroke. On the other hand, the more HDL cholesterol (high-density lipoprotein) present in the body, the lower the risk of coronary heart disease.

Hormones like estrogen also influence the synthesis of blood serum cholesterol. Consequently, being overweight for a woman may pose additional risks to health in that fat cells produce more estrogen which can lead to faulty cholesterol metabolism and even tumor formation. Some of the cholesterol factors that increase the risk of developing heart disease are:

- elevated total blood cholesterol levels greater that 200 mg per deciliter
- elevated LDL cholesterol levels greater than 130 mg per deciliter
- HDL cholesterol levels that create a ratio of total cholesterol to HDL cholesterol greater than 4.5 to 1
- obesity
- fat stores which accumulate above the waist

Reducing dietary fat is the one most effective way to lower blood cholesterol and the risk of heart disease. The obesity factor is emerging as much more important than previously thought. New findings strongly suggest that even a relatively small amount of excess weight (between ten and twenty pounds) can predispose an individual to the development of heart disease. For those of us who suffer from a "fat imbalance," a condition where we store more fat than we burn, it is often a matter of life or death to lose fat in order to protect our arteries and hearts.

PRESCRIPTION FOR WEIGHT LOSS

We know that lowering fat content in our diets and exercising are important, but state of the art research in the area of weight loss has also discovered that with the addition of certain supplements and nutrients, the process of decreasing the amount of fat we process and boosting the amount of fat we burn can be expedited.

CHAPTER 4

NATURAL SUBSTANCES THAT METABOLIZE FAT

This chapter will look at various natural supplements that affect fats by either absorbing them after ingestion, breaking them down more efficiently, or discouraging their storage as excess weight. Several compounds exist in nature which can serve to expedite the burning of fat. Today, science is concentrating on orchestrating a pharmaceutical compound capable of neutralizing fats after they have been consumed.

Most weight reducing strategies have to confront the problem of burning already stored fat. Usually we become overweight and then go about the business of trying to remedy the problem. Despite the truth of the adage that "an ounce of prevention is worth a pound of cure," most of us continue to eat high-fats diets, waiting until something serious happens before we take action.

As most of us know, the process of dieting is grueling and can leave us discouraged, fatigued and more fat susceptible. Dieting attempts to undo what has already biologically occurred and involves reversing the metabolic process to a great degree. It's much easier to prevent a fat buildup than to reverse the damage that carrying extra fat stores can cause.

Weight Gain Begins in the Stomach

The body begins to digest lipids in the stomach and intestines, where it is eventually absorbed into the bloodstream and metabolized and stored by the liver, or used as a fuel source for immediate energy. During their bloodstream journey, fats can become trapped in the veins and arteries, especially if they have sustained any type of free radical damage. A damaged artery contains rough spots which can snag lipids. Ideally, if we could neutralize fat after it has entered our stomach, we could spare our physiological systems from having to deal with that fat.

Lipid Calories vs. Carbohydrate and Protein Calories

The human body is designed to stockpile fat very easily. This tendency is related to innate mechanisms intended to protect us against starvation or the threat of a diminished food supply. Fat cells provide extra fuel which can be utilized if necessary to sustain life. The negative aspect is that fats are readily converted to pounds. When we eat more fat than the body requires (and most of us do), that fat is stored. "Fat packets" settle on the hips, the waist or the thighs, not to mention the upper arms and back. Fats can also be stored around organs, like the heart, as well as inside veins and arteries, a potentially fatal situation. Laboratory tests which have taken a test tube of blood from an individual who has eaten a double cheeseburger, french fries and a thick milk shake have found that the blood becomes a milky pink color due to the infusion of fat from the digestive system. This fat circulates through the system until it is either burned or stored.

Carbohydrates and proteins require more complicated digestive processes to convert and store their energy than fat does. Calories from carbohydrates and proteins are usually burned and thrown off as heat (thermogenesis). Naturally, overeating proteins and carbohydrates can result in weight gain, but the body has to work harder to convert those nutrients to fat stores. It actually takes more energy to change these nutrients into adipose tissue (body fat) than to convert dietary fat to adipose tissue. It takes about 5 percent of the energy content of dietary fat to convert it to body fat. But it takes 20 to 25 percent of the energy content of carbohydrate and protein to convert them to body fat.

CHITOSAN: A FAT ABSORBER

Any day now, FDA-approved drugs that block fat from being absorbed in the gut will emerge as the new weight reduction replacement to the now forbidden phen-fen. Orlistat is the generic name of a synthetic compound which binds to fat, making it undigestible. Ironically, a natural fiber-like substance which does precisely the same thing has been available through health food distributors for some time. It is called chitosan—a natural compound which has proven its efficacy in keeping fat from being assimilated in the digestive tract.

Chitosan is a fat-binding agent found in the chitin of crab and shrimp shells. It has the ability to prevent fat absorption in the stomach by attracting fat and binding with lipid molecules, making them too large to pass through the walls of the gastrointestinal tract. As a result, they are eliminated in an undigested state.

Chitosan has been used for about seventeen years in the detoxification of water. When chitosan is spread over the surface of water, it literally absorbs greases, oils, heavy metals and other potentially toxic substances. Like a fat magnet, it attracts these biohazardous substances to such an extent that a residue forms on the top of the water and can be easily scraped off. Water purification plants throughout the nation use chitosan for this purpose. This indicated to scientists that chitosan could selectively absorb fats even in a water medium. It was especially relevant that chitosan absorbed only the fats and not the water.

What Exactly is Chitosan?

Chitosan is a natural product derived from chitin, a polysaccharide found in the exoskeleton of shellfish like shrimp or crabs. While it has been in existence for millennia, its current form has only recently been synthesized. Technically speaking, chitosan is a naturally occurring substance that is chemically similar the plant fiber cellulose. Like plant fibers, chitosan possesses many of the same properties as fiber, however, unlike plant fiber, it has the ability to significantly bind fat, acting like a sponge in the digestive tract.

The process of synthesizing chitosan involves taking the shells of shrimp or crabs, grinding them to a fine powder, and then deacetylating this powder. This refers to the removal of specific chemicals so that the remaining compound is more active in its ability to soak up fats. Like some plant fibers, chitosan is not digestible, therefore it has no caloric value. No matter how much chitosan you ingest, its calorie count remains at zero. This is an very important property for any weight-loss product.

How Does Chitosan Work?

Chitosan affects fat in the stomach before it has a chance to become metabolized. Chitosan dissolves in the stomach and converts to a gel which captures fat, thereby preventing its absorption and storage. A "grease ball" of excess fat that is too large to be metabolized is created, and both the chitosan and the unmetabolized fat are excreted in the stool. In this way chitosan renders fat useless to the body. Simply stated, chitosan:

- binds excess fat molecules and fatty acids
- binds dietary cholesterol
- reduces the absorption of all of the above
- can function as a non-digestible dietary fiber
- correlates with improved cardiovascular health

Chitosan: A Form Of Fiber

After years of fiber hype, most of us are well aware of the profound benefits that fiber has for human health and longevity. Fiber is considered a dieter's best friend. The *International Journal of Obesity* has stated that adding dietary fiber to a low-fat diet can help reduce hunger and increase the number of bowel movements; two actions which greatly enhance weight loss. Fiber has also been linked to slower rises in blood glucose which profoundly affect how we store excess calories and when we feel hungry.

Chitosan is a positively charged fiber that binds to negatively charged fatty acids. Technically speaking, chitosan is *lipophilic*, meaning that it is chemically attracted to fat. Most fibers are *hydrophilic*, which means they repel fat and attract water. Psyllium, for example, is used for its bulk-forming action. This type of fiber absorbs water and is easily passed through the intestine, helping to maintain a normal stool.

While chitosan possesses many of the same benefits as plant fibers like psyllium, it can also inactivate fats. For this reason, combining chitosan with fibers like psyllium is highly recommended and only serves to further support the weight-loss process. Chitosan will bind the fat and psyllium will speed its journey through the intestines to be expelled.

Chitosan is considered a crude fiber that can also improve the bulk of the stool. Stool samples tested in people who have taken chitosan confirm that an increased absorption of fat has occurred. Under optimal conditions, chitosan can bind four to five times its weight with all the lipid aggregates tested.[8] (*Note:* This assessment was made without the addition of ascorbic acid which potentiates this action even further. Studies in Helsinki have shown that individuals taking chitosan lost as average of 8 percent of their body weight in a four week period.[9])

Fiber advocates recommend a diet calorically fueled with between 10 and 20 percent fat and 35 to 45 grams of fiber. Unfortunately, most of us—no matter how good our intentions—

will not be able to sustain this type of diet. A diet that reduces fat intake from 20 to 30 percent and increases fiber to 20 or 30 grams is much more feasible in controlling weight, avoiding artery disease and promoting good colon health.

Taking chitosan prior to eating a meal can make dietary fat goals attainable and promote a number of desirable health benefits. Because obesity ranks among the top ten diseases (which are almost all related to obesity), the notion of a safe, health promoting fat blocker is desirable. Weight-loss programs usually involve a lifestyle that many of us can never incorporate. While chitosan is not the magic answer to maintaining a youthful figure, it is a very powerful dietary complement which can facilitate what might otherwise be unattainable. Lowering the amount of fat we eat, exercising more and making sure we get enough fiber seems to be the winning combination for health and longevity. Chitosan serves as a valuable vehicle for attaining optimal nutrition and health.

Other Therapeutic Benefits of Chitosan

CHOLESTEROL CONTROL

- Chitosan has the very unique ability to lower LDL cholesterol (the bad kind) while boosting HDL cholesterol (the good kind).[10]
- Laboratory tests performed on rats showed that "chitosan depresses serum and liver cholesterol levels in cholesterol-fed rats without affecting performance, organ weight or the nature of the feces."[11]
- Japanese researchers conclude that chitosan "appears to be an effective hypocholesterolemic agent."[12] In other words, it can effectively lower blood serum cholesterol levels without apparent side effects.
- A study presented in the *American Journal of Clinical Nutrition* found that chitosan is as effective as cholestryramine (a cholesterol-lowering drug) in controlling blood

serum cholesterol without the deleterious side effects typical of cholestryramine.[13]

- Chitosan has been shown to decrease blood cholesterol levels by 66.2 percent.[14]
- Chitosan effectively lowered cholesterol absorption more than guar gum or cellulose.[15]
- Laboratory test results indicated that a 7.5 percent chitosan formula maintained adequate cholesterol levels in rats, despite a dramatic increase in the intake of cholesterol.[16]

CHITOSAN AND HIGH BLOOD PRESSURE

Some clinical studies have found that chitosan works as a antihypertensive agent and lowered blood pressure in male subjects which were fed a high salt diet.[17] Chitosan also has the ability to decrease blood levels of chloride which influences the activity of an angiotensin converting enzyme. Angiotensin is vital to the maintenance of normal blood pressure.[18]

CHITOSAN, CALCIUM ABSORPTION AND BONE HEALTH

Clinical tests have found that chitosan enhances the bioavailability of calcium which means that its absorbability is increased.[19] The more calcium available, the better bone quality will be. The prevention of osteoporosis depends on continual supplies of absorbable calcium. Chitosan has actually been used as a supplementary food for osteoporosis. Apparently, chitosan activates certain macrophages, an action that boosts the metabolism of bone and expedites the absorption of calcium in the intestine.[20]

ASCORBIC ACID AND CHITOSAN

When certain substances are added to chitosan, its remarkable fat-binding ability can be significantly enhanced. Ascorbic acid is one of these substances. Ascorbic acid, a source of vitamin C, serves to enhance the absorbability of lipids. Clinical studies verify that supplementing chitosan with ascorbic acid results in less fat digestion and absorption in the intestines than with chitosan alone.[21] In fact, the addition of ascorbic acid almost doubles chitosan's effectiveness as a fat blocker.

CITRIC ACID AND CHITOSAN

Citric acid also boosts the swelling action of chitosan, thereby providing increased satiety and appetite suppression. Combining citric acid with chitosan resulted in an overall reduction in food intake. Using *Garcinia cambogia* is recommended because it contains hydroxycitric acid (HCA). This form of citric acid inhibits the liver's ability to make fats out of carbohydrates. Consequently, carbohydrates are converted to glycogen stores, not fat stores, which means that the body has a better reserve of fuel and stamina is increased.

How To Take Chitosan

Because chitosan binds with fats, it should not be taken with certain lipid-based vitamins, minerals or medications. The best way to take chitosan is just prior to a high-fat meal, usually lunch or dinner. In order to avoid any type of nutrient deficiency, take other supplements in the morning when chitosan is not used.

If you decide to take a chitosan-containing supplement, make sure to follow its dosage suggestions. The amount of chitosan you take usually depends on how fatty your meal is. Whenever taking any form of fiber, drinking at least eight glasses of water per day is highly recommended.

Safety Issues: Chitosan is considered safe and is environmentally friendly. Other than its fat-binding action, chitosan remains virtually inactive in the human body. It is low in toxicity and allergic properties. Studies in which rats consumed a diet of up to 15 percent chitosan showed no toxic side effects. You should not take chitosan if you have any kind of shellfish allergy or are pregnant or breast feeding. If you are taking medication of any kind, check with your physician before using chitosan.

FAT METABOLIZERS

This section discusses natural compounds which help to breakdown fat molecules, thereby allowing the body to more easily burn them off as energy. Several compounds exist in nature which have proven their ability to either speed up the metabolism of lipids or to discourage their storage. Thermogenic compounds which convert calories to heat will be discussed in the following section.

Citrin or Hydroxycitric Acid (*Garcinia cambogia*)

Hydroxycitric acid (HCA) is found in the tropical rain forest herb *Garcinia cambogia* and can actually inhibit the conversion of carbohydrates to fat by the liver, thereby boosting thermogenesis.[22] This action is extremely beneficial to anyone who is attempting to facilitate weight loss. HCA converts carbohydrates into glycogen stores rather than into fat. (Glycogen refers to glucose that has been stored as one of the body's main sources of readily available energy.) This remarkable effect enhances stamina and builds important energy reserves. Moreover, when glycogen stores are created, the appestat center of the brain creates a feeling of satiety or fullness, inhibiting the desire to overeat. People who have trouble controlling their weight often suffer from the inability to store glycogen properly. As a result, their brain is continually stimulated to send hunger signals, resulting in unnecessary eating and weight gain.

HCA is also thought to have the ability to actually alter the way in which fat cells accumulate.. Clinical tests support the ability of HCA to decrease body fat without losing body protein or lean muscle mass.[23] In addition, it works to suppress the appetite if taken thirty minutes before a meal. It can also lower cholesterol levels.[24] Doses vary from 500 to 1500 mg per day.

Safety Issues: HCA is generally recognized as safe with no known toxicity. Just make sure to drink plenty of water when taking HCA in order to expedite the removal of fat from the body. Citric acid or vitamin C can also contribute to its action.

Choline

Choline is involved in the transport of fats and cholesterol and greatly contributes to the body's ability to digest fats. Choline is a lipotropic agent in that it prevents the buildup of fats in the liver and other body tissues. Lecithin is a natural source of choline and enables fats like cholesterol to be flushed from the body. In this way lecithin contributes to good arterial health—it discourages fatty build-up which can cause heart disease and hypertension. It also plays an important role in hormone regulation, which is essential to stabilizing weight and appetite. Dosages of choline can vary from 500 to 3000 mg per day.

Safety Issues: Lecithin and choline are considered safe supplements if not taken in high doses. Very high doses of lecithin or choline can cause nausea, diarrhea or depression. The amounts of choline usually included in thermogenic formulas should not cause these kinds of reactions.

Essential Fatty Acids

Taking an essential fatty acid (EFA) supplement such as flaxseed oil is recommended as an addition to any thermogenic formula. EFAs exert a significant lipid-lowering effect. It is important to realize that with all the emphasis we put on the perils of dietary fats, the body must have a certain amount of beneficial fat in order to function, and even to lose weight. Cases studies confirm that weight loss plateaus experienced by certain groups of women on diets were broken with the addition of flaxseed oil. It is believed that oils like flaxseed actually stimulate the brown-fat stores where fat is burned.

The hormone known as prostaglandin E1 may play an important role in activating brown fat stores. This substance is made from fatty acids found in flaxseeds. Scientists theorize that people who stay perpetually thin may have very active brown-fat stores while obese individuals have dormant brown fat.[25] In short, EFAs which include omega-3 oils have the ability to boost thermogenesis by increasing the metabolic rate. They also help to eliminate excess fluid from the body.[26]

Safety Issues: Flaxseed oil is considered safe, but fish oil sources of omega-3 fatty acids should be avoided by diabetics.

DHEA

DHEA inhibits the action of a specific enzyme which contributes to fat production. Research supports an inverse relationship between low DHEA blood levels and obesity.[27] Not only does DHEA appear to step up the fat-burning process (thermogenesis), it decreases the desire to eat. One study found that DHEA increased serotonin levels in the brain which resulted in less food cravings.[28] Apparently, serotonin levels profoundly affect our moods, carbohydrate cravings, food intake and body fat. Several new studies have discovered that a desire to eat is not always based on true hunger. Frequently, it is neurochemistry that determines when, what and why we eat. A persistent feeling of being hungry or not satisfied can be inhibited by serotonin release within brain cells. DHEA works to stimulate the release of serotonin in the hypothalamus region of the brain, which in turn reduces our desire to eat.

A 1995 study concluded that women who received DHEA as hormone replacement therapy decreased their food intake. DHEA significantly decreased the desire to eat and was considered an appetite suppressant.[29] Another recent study found that rats consumed a great deal more food after DHEA supplementation was stopped. "Upon removing dietary DHEA, rats immediately consumed significantly more food than while on the DHEA supplemented diets."[30] Another study concluded that DHEA administration has an antiobesity effect.[31]

It is interesting to note that the presence of fat may contribute to the promotion of more fat by adversely effecting DHEA levels. In 1991 a group of researchers concluded that people with severe obesity are unable to increase their natural DHEA levels due to their high percentage of body fat. It is thought that this faulty mechanism contributes to the progressive accumulation of more fat and creates a vicious cycle.[32]

DHEA's involvement in thermogenesis has been referred to as "energy wastage."[33] "Energy waste is thought to be one of the ways that DHEA reduces body weight . . . Obesity and diabetes are characterized by high levels of gluconeogenesis, occurring in spite of increased levels of insulin . . . DHEA reduced gluconeogenesis."[34] Unquestionably, the implications of DHEA therapy for obesity are significant and require further exploration. Initial test results suggest the viability of using DHEA to help treat and prevent obesity.

Safety Issues: DHEA should not be used by pregnant or nursing women or anyone with hormonally-related cancers. The effects of long-term use of DHEA are still unresearched.

Pyruvate

Pyruvate is a natural compound which has been found to significantly impact not only weight loss, but also fat loss.[35] Pyruvate is naturally found in the body and is essential for the proper metabolism of nutrients into energy. It is also found in foods such as some cheeses and red apples. At this writing, pyruvate is enjoying significant popularity as a weight-loss aid. A recent study reported that "subjects fed pyruvate showed a greater weight and fat loss than the group fed simply a low-energy diet. The group receiving pyruvate demonstrated an average of 37 percent greater weight loss and 48 percent greater fat loss compared to the placebo group."[36] Another plus about pyruvate is that it is thought to increase resting metabolic rate and increase fat utilization.

Dosage: Dosage issues are still unresolved although the general consensus is that anything lower than five grams or more than twelve grams is not recommended.

Safety Issues: Pyruvate has caused diarrhea, slight nausea and intestinal gas in some individuals, but is considered safe if used in appropriate doses. It should not be used by pregnant or lactating women. The effects of long term use of pyruvate are still unresearched.

DMAE

DMAE (dimethylaminoethanol) is a compound which, among other things, is considered a neurostimulant. It has been used for everything from memory and learning enhancement to increased stamina. It is most commonly used as a mild stimulant which boosts energy without interfering with sleep patterns. DMAE is believed to contribute to increased mental awareness and stamina without the significant side effects of caffeine or amphetamine drugs. The hangover effect typically associated with other stimulant drugs does not occur with DMAE therapy. Neither does DMAE produce the mood slumps and fatigue which occur when other stimulant drugs are discontinued.

In relation to weight loss, DMAE contributes to heightened metabolism and thermogenesis by boosting energy levels as well as helping reduce body fat stores. It is thought to work in tandem with herbs like ephedra to help maximize thermogenesis, although no clinical studies supporting this action exist. DMAE can be found in certain seafood and is naturally present in very minute quantities in brain tissue. It is considered a nutritional supplement and is available in capsules, liquids or powdered forms. If using the liquid form of DMAE, refrigeration is required to preserve potency. DMAE may also be added to various formulas designed to boost energy, fight fatigue or burn fat

Safety Issues: DMAE can have significant side effects if taken in large quantities or if overused. Insomnia, headaches and muscle stiffness above the neck or in the legs indicate that DMAE dosages are too high. While there are no adverse reactions to DMAE on record, anyone with manic-depressive illness or epilepsy should not use DMAE without the approval of their physician. The rule with DMAE is to begin with the smallest possible dose.

Coenzyme Q10

A deficiency of coenzyme Q10 has been associated with obesity. Recent studies have indicated that this micronutrient may be more vital to metabolic processes than previously thought. By supplying the body with adequate levels of coenzyme Q10, some researchers believe that improved lipid metabolism and enhanced cellular control of fat stores will result. Studies suggest that coenzyme Q10 may be intimately linked to thermogenesis in brown adipose tissue and that it may help to regulate and boost thermogenic activity. Consider the following quote regarding a study on the effects of coenzyme Q10 and obesity: ". . . the obvious fact remains that people who were deficient in coenzyme Q10 were able to shed more pounds when their coenzyme Q10 levels were boosted than overweight people who had no coenzyme Q10 deficiency."[37] What this study implies is that obese individuals should have their coenzyme Q10 levels checked and corrected in order to facilitate the burning of fat.

Chapter 5

Thermogenic Agents: Converting Calories to Heat

Thermogenics, or the burning of fats, involves certain compounds which have the ability to rev up the fat furnace by restoring brown fat activity. As mentioned earlier, thermogenics focuses on weight loss through the correction of fat metabolism rather than on caloric restriction or brain chemistry manipulation. Some of the best natural weight-loss supplements which base their design on thermogenics combine a number of natural ingredients that work synergistically to create the optimal metabolic effect. In addition, some formulas provide certain nutrients which further expedite the process of converting fat to energy. In order to most effectively accomplish thermogenesis, compounds should be assembled which help to curb cravings, discourage the storage of calories as fat, and help to stabilize blood sugar levels, a function intrinsically linked to the sensation of hunger.

When combined with a normal diet and adequate water replenishment, thermogenic substances can significantly enhance our ability to lose weight. Boosting the caloric furnace without compromising stamina is also crucial to successful fat metabolism.

THERMOGENESIS: A DEFINITION

Thermogenics is an area of weight management which has recently received a great deal of attention within scientific circles. Some experts refer to thermogenics as the most significant discovery in weight management research to occur in the last thirty years. Why each of us have different thermogenic capacities is currently under research. This booklet discusses a number of natural compounds which "stoke the furnace" of this metabolic process, resulting in quicker and more efficient weight loss. As previously mentioned, the word *thermogenesis* literally means "the creation of heat." When we create heat, we are burning excess calories in order to maintain our weight or, in some cases, actually decrease it. Any substance which stimulates the resting metabolic rate (RMR) and results in raising the body temperature is called a thermogenic agent. When this biological process ensues, noradrenalin production is also increased and serves to stimulate the breakdown of fat.

A good number of health care practitioners believe that correcting or enhancing the metabolic process, which determines how we convert food to fat or to fuel is a safer and much more efficient way to attack obesity. The term *thermogenics* refers to a relatively new science which explores ways in which metabolism converts dietary calories to heat rather than to energy or fat. Among the many methodologies of weight loss, targeting the metabolic furnace and enhancing its ability to burn fat will be the focus of this discussion.

The science of thermogenics holds the key to safe and effective weight loss because it focuses on the biological processes which burn off fat rather than targeting the appestat center of the brain or manipulating food consumption. It is crucial to remember that the safety and efficacy of thermogenics depends on using the proper combination of compounds in recommended proportions and dosages.

Storing Fat: A Survival Mechanism

The body is designed to store fat in order to sustain us during periods when nourishment may decrease. It is vital to remember that each person has a unique body which operates at its own programmed metabolic rate. It is also important to keep in mind that storing fat is a natural function. Fat stores are designed to protect our organs and ward off starvation. The widespread notion that you will gain weight if you consume too many calories and fail to exercise enough is a rather simplistic explanation of what is a very complex and individualized biological function. The truth is that if we deprive ourselves of calories it can initiate what is referred to as a "starvation response," causing metabolic processes to slow down. This survival response causes our bodies to cling to our fat stores more tenaciously than ever and to efficiently convert what we eat to fat, in anticipation of another bout with food deprivation.

Brown Fat: A Good Thing

Over the last few years, scientists have discovered the existence of relatively small pockets of brown fatty tissue, also referred to as BAT (brown adipose tissue), in specific regions of the body. This brown fat has the distinctive ability to burn excess calories from dietary sources and to contribute to the burning of stored fat. Chemically speaking, brown fat contains a unique protein which causes calories to be burned off as heat. Burning calories during thermogenesis helps to prevent fat storage. BAT contains tiny molecules of protein which have the distinct ability to interfere with the biochemical process which causes calories to be used as energy in other tissues. What this means is that when brown fat is stimulated properly, calories are continually converted to heat and white fat stores are reduced. The heat simply radiates off and quickly dissipates.

Several theories suggest that under certain conditions brown fat no longer performs its thermogenic function and as a result pounds accumulate. When the thermogenic mechanism of brown fat is impaired, our bodies conserve fuel by increasing our fat stores rather than burning off any excess calories we consume. Because of this, when BAT thermogenesis is faulty, obesity may result. As unfair as this might seem, someone with low brown fat stores may convert 30 percent less of their caloric intake into heat as compared with lean individuals. Heredity, mid-life physiological changes or excessive dieting can contribute to a loss of BAT activity.

Dieting deserves a word here because, ironically, anytime we drastically reduce our caloric intake in order to shed a few pounds, we set a number of biochemical events into motion which make brown fat less active. In a very efficient manner, the body conserves fat and stores it even more readily than before in anticipation of a threat to its fuel supply. Consequently, metabolism slows and though fat may be initially lost, it is quickly replaced when normal eating patterns resume. Low-calorie diets serve to completely defeat the purpose of weight loss because they cause the body to turn down the caloric furnace.

What To Look For in a Thermogenic Formula

Finding a reliable and effective thermogenic formula is the key to weight loss success. Ideally, such a blend should include natural substances which:

- suppress the appetite
- stimulate the burning of fat
- promote regularity
- support the adrenal glands
- control carbohydrate cravings
- provide energy
- form lean muscle mass
- boost elimination of fluids

Combinations that include supplements which accomplish these aims will be most effective. The remainder of this chapter discusses individual substances which accomplish a variety of biochemical actions designed to augment and support thermogenesis.

MAJOR COMPOUNDS FOUND IN THERMOGENIC FORMULAS

Ephedra

Chinese ephedra, also known as *ma huang,* is an ancient herb which promotes the breakdown of fat through the thermogenic process. It is the only plant stimulant which promotes brown fat thermogenesis and is the single most important element in any thermogenic formula. Many cultures have long used this herb and consider it safe if taken appropriately. Ephedra has credible and impressive thermogenic properties which prompt the body to look to a fat source rather than to muscle protein. While it does not suppress the appetite, ephedra can reduce cravings in that whenever fat burning takes place, insulin levels drop and hunger is better controlled.

The pharmacology of ephedra revolves around a compound called ephedrine, or pseudoephedrine. Several recent studies published in the *International Journal of Obesity* concluded that ephedrine (the primary chemical constituent of ephedra) is a thermogenic agent which can enhance one's ability to burn fat by increasing the resting metabolic rate and by boosting the activity of brown adipose tissue (BAT).[38]

Ephedra is considered a botanical stimulant and its action is similar to that of adrenalin, although as a compound, it is much less potent. Because of its stimulatory effect, it enhances energy output by boosting circulation and increasing the force of heart muscle contraction. As a result, more oxygen is supplied to muscle tissue, and muscle performance is increased. Ephedra mildly stimulates the central nervous system and can cause stimulant-like effects. Because it can raise blood pressure, it is not recommended for anyone suffering from heart disease or hypertension.

Several studies support the use of ephedrine for weight loss. When used in appropriate dosages, the biochemical mechanics of ephedrine step up the breakdown of fatty tissue for fuel.

Apparently, ephedrine stimulates the sympathetic nervous system which, in turn, boosts thermogenesis. In one study, ephedrine was able to initiate a 14 percent reduction in body weight and a 42 percent loss of body fat.[39] When other complementary compounds were added to ephedrine, the results were even more impressive.[40] A very recent study found that ephedra did indeed activate the activity of BAT and was particularly effective when combined with other agents.[41]

Practically speaking, taking ephedra alone to achieve weight loss is not recommended. While test results support its ability to boost the metabolism of fat, the amount of ephedra required to produce desirable results is too high. But when ephedra is combined with caffeine and salicylic acid, its effect is significantly enhanced, making it possible to attain weight loss with acceptable therapeutic levels of each compound. For this reason, searching out formulas that are properly balanced is essential.

Safety Issues: Ephedra has received a stamp of approval by the FDA and is considered a safe supplement if taken in recommended dosages. It is routinely included in hundreds of over-the-counter medications for colds and allergies. It is quickly excreted from the body and *if used properly* has a good safety record.[42] Individuals suffering from heart disease, anxiety attacks, high blood pressure, diabetes, adrenal disease, thyroid disease or prostate disorders should not take products containing ephedrine. People who are taking antidepressants or drugs for high blood pressure should not use ephedra. While clinical studies have found ephedra to be safe during pregnancy, it is not recommended for nursing or pregnant women.

Possible side effects of ephedra supplementation include insomnia, anxiety, increased heart rate and blood pressure, skin flushing or tingling and nausea. Significant side effects are usually associated with large doses of ephedra. Recently, ephedra received a great deal of media attention due to incidents where extremely high doses were taken to achieve an amphetamine-like "high." Abusing any herb or over-the-counter medication in this way could be life-threatening. Ephedra should be taken in combination with other ingredients designed to both buffer and temper its effects. (*Note:* Consuming caffeine containing beverages with ephedra may result in a jittery feeling or indicate a sensitivity to stimulant agents. If the feeling persists, doses should be lowered or stopped altogether. Check with your physician.)

Compounds Which Potentiate Ephedrine

While several studies have confirmed the ability of ephedrine alone to stimulate weight loss, adding certain compounds to the ephedra mix creates a much more efficient thermogenic formula. In order to achieve desired results using ephedra alone, dosages fall into a range most professionals do not feel comfortable with. Moreover, test results have suggested that taking ephedrine alone is not as effective in stimulating weight loss as compared to combination blends. By adding specific compounds to ephedra, its thermogenic effect becomes attainable with much lower doses. Aspirin, salicylate herbs like white willow, caffeine-containing plants and other herbs such as guarana, kola nut, yerba mate enhance the thermogenic effects of ephedra.

White Willow

White willow is a natural herbal source of salicylates and is often added to ephedra. In 1827, a French chemist named Leroux was able to extract the principle pharmacological compound from white willow which he found worked as an effective pain reliever. He called this substance salicin, after the willow genus known as salix. Salicin is converted to salicylic acid, the primary molecule which comprises aspirin after ingestion.

The salicylate content of white willow is believed by some to mimic the effect of aspirin with ephedra. White willow compounds can accomplish the same potentiating effect as aspirin by contributing to increased body temperature due to the burning of fatty deposits. Some professionals believe that only aspirin will accomplish this effect, while others find the salicylate contribution of white willow both safe and effective.

Numerous clinical studies involving both animals and humans have confirmed the impressive benefits of ephedra in promoting weight loss and stimulating a number of thermogenic mechanisms.[43] Clinical findings disclose that adding an aspirin, which contains salicylates, works to further potentiate the thermogenic effect of ephedrine.[44] Studies involving both lean and overweight women with this combination found that adding aspirin to ephedrine raised the resting metabolic rate by 0.21 and 0.19 kilocalories per minute.[45]

Safety Issues: Taking white willow may cause some gastrointestinal upset if taken on an empty stomach. In addition, white willow may interfere with the absorption of iron if they are taken together. Anyone who is allergic to salicylates should avoid this herb. White willow should not be used during viral infections, especially chicken pox.

Guarana

Guarana is classified as a methylxanthine herb and is often used in thermogenic formulas that feature ephedra. Its chemical constituents make it the perfect complementary drug to ephedra. Guarana contains natural theophylline and caffeine which when added to ephedra greatly enhance total body fat loss.[46] This duo significantly stimulates increased metabolism and fat-cell breakdown.

Guarana is considered by some to be a preferable plant source of caffeine, which has impressive thermogenic properties when mixed with ephedrine and theophylline. Several studies support the safe addition of these compounds to ephedra and indicate that their presence greatly enhances the basal metabolic rate and diet-related thermogenesis.[47]

Dosages: Look for combinations which can supply between 500 and 1000 milligrams of ephedra per day. The addition of white willow and herbs like guarana serve to enhance the thermogenic properties of any ephedra-based weight loss formula. Recommended dosages should be taken at least thirty minutes prior to meals.

Safety Issues: No records of toxicity has been recorded regarding guarana, which is classified by the FDA as "generally regarded as safe." Certain side effects can occur and include insomnia, dizziness, increased heart rate, increased blood pressure and tremors. In tests using guarana and ephedra side effects diminished and the long term effect on blood pressure was positive as it dropped in response to weight loss that occurred.[48] It is important not to take excessive doses of ephedra and guarana combinations. High doses are not required to achieve desired results.

Green Tea Extract

Green tea contains plant caffeine and theophylline. It is also rich in flavonoid compounds which have significant antioxidant properties, including catechin. Green tea helps to protect against cancer, lowers blood cholesterol levels, and inhibits the formation of blood clots. It has also proven itself as a valuable weight loss aid which also boosts energy levels. When used in conjunction with ephedra or other weight loss supplements, it promotes the burning of fat and helps to normalize blood sugar and insulin levels, which can help suppress abnormal hunger and food cravings. It is also believed that green tea may prevent the absorption of dietary fat through the walls of the gastrointestinal tract. Green tea should not be used alone, but in formulas designed to stimulate weight loss the complex chemistry of green tea adds a number of therapeutic actions.

Safety Issues: Green tea should not be used in large amounts by pregnant or nursing women. Anyone suffering from a heart disorder, irregular heartbeat or anxiety attacks should not take green tea unless advised to do so by their physician.

Kola Nut, Bissy Nut, Goo Roo Nut, or Yerba Mate

Any one or a combination of these herbs may be added to ephedra-based thermogenic formulas. They are natural plant sources of caffeine which has been proven to boost the thermogenic ability of ephedra.

NUTRIENTS THAT SUPPORT THE ADRENAL GLANDS

The process of thermogenesis taxes the adrenal glands, so it is important to provide adrenal support with certain supplements. Through supplementation adrenal exhaustion can be prevented. In addition, taking a two to three day break from any thermogenic regimen is recommended in order to provide the body with an "adrenal rest period." Some experts believe that anyone who feels exhausted while taking a thermogenic formula may be suffering from adrenal insufficiency. If this is the case, building up the adrenal glands before starting a thermogenic protocol is recommended.

Vitamin B12 (Dibencozide)

The process of thermogenesis utilizes hormones which are produced by the adrenal glands. As a result, the adrenals can become fatigued. The addition of vitamin B12 helps to nourish and support the adrenal glands. In addition, B12 helps to regulate the metabolism of carbohydrates and is believed to support the thermogenic function of brown adipose tissue (BAT).

Licorice Root

Licorice root works to protect and support the adrenal glands which can become overworked during by thermogenic agents. Frequently, during periods of stress or if the production of certain adrenal hormones is stimulated, the adrenal glands fail to adequately manage the biological needs of the body. The chemical constituents of licorice help to reverse this effect and prevent adrenal fatigue. Licorice compounds have the ability to maintain normal electrolyte balance in body tissues, thus enabling adrenocortical hormones to circulate and retain their activity for longer periods of time.[49] In addition, licorice helps to regulate low blood sugar which can result from poor adrenal function.[50] Deglycyrrhizinated licorice (DGL) is the preferred form.

Safety Issues: Licorice is considered a safe herb if not taken in large amounts over an extended time period. In combination formulas which include licorice, its dosage is usually much too small to cause concern; however, licorice should not be used by pregnant women, anyone with diabetes, glaucoma, high blood pressure, heart disease, or stroke. Prolonged use of licorice (more than seven consecutive days) can result in elevated blood pressure in persons who are predisposed to hypertension. It can cause sodium retention and potassium depletion if used in large enough doses. Potassium supplementation is sometimes recommended when taking licorice. DGL forms of licorice have less side effects.

Ginseng

This ancient herb helps to support and restore adrenal function, especially during times of mental or physiological stress. It is also believed to contribute to lipid breakdown.

THERMOGENIC WEIGHT LOSS

Time Factors

While the time required for weight loss with thermogenic formulas can vary with each person, the process usually takes several weeks. It is believed that individuals with low brown-fat stores will lose weight at a slower rate. Remember that taking thermogenic agents may actually help to increase brown-fat stores, thus increasing one's ability to lose weight with continued use. People who suffer from adrenal or thyroid diseases may not be candidates for thermogenic weight loss and should check with their physicians. Anyone with hypothyroidism may want to add an acceptable exercise program to their thermogenic protocol with the approval of their physician. All things considered, thermogenic weight loss can be accomplished in a relatively short time, depending on the amount of weight loss desired.

The Exercise Component

One of the possible bonuses of thermogenic compounds is their ability to enhance the weight reducing effects of exercise. Some experts believe that exercising too soon after taking a thermogenic formula is not as effective as waiting from two to four hours. This reasoning is based on the notion that exercise raises body temperature, thereby interfering with the thermogenic release of heat from calories. Exercise should be planned during time intervals when thermogenic activity is at its lowest.

Guidelines

- Take only recommended doses of any thermogenic formulas. Remember that more does not mean better.
- Thermogenic formulas can be taken with or between meals, but it is best to take them at the same time each day. Consistency is the key.
- Most people do not consume thermogenic agents past 3:00 pm to avoid insomnia.
- Do not take any thermogenic formula without allowing for time periods where the body can rest from adrenal stimulation. On for four, off for three is sometimes recommended.
- If you experience any adverse side effects, either lower the

dosage or stop altogether. Always check with your physician before beginning a thermogenic program for weight loss.

Contraindications: Anyone with heart disease, prostate disease, thyroid disease, high blood pressure, diabetes or adrenal disease should not use thermogenic agents without their doctor's approval. Pregnant or nursing women should not use these compounds in that they may stimulate the infant's central nervous system. (*Note:* Mild constipation can occur with thermogenic compounds. Drink plenty of water and eat fiber-rich foods to help to alleviate this effect. Herbs like cascara sagrada can also ease constipation and keep the bowels regular.)

Taking a good thermogenic formula can result is some very positive and often unexpected side effects. Frequently people who are on a thermogenic protocol will also experience:

- increased mental alertness
- better productivity and performance
- boosted energy levels
- improved asthma/ allergy symptoms
- lower cholesterol levels
- alleviation of depression
- feeling of well-being
- blood pressure drop with long-term use
- less interest in eating

The science of thermogenics holds significant promise for the weight management. It focuses on how the body utilizes dietary calories to produce heat rather than calories stored as fat or used as energy. Unquestionably, specific natural compounds exist which facilitate this metabolic phenomenon. Several thermogenic formulas are now available and should be assessed for their ingredients and reliability.

Anyone who experiences any type of adverse side effects with any thermogenic product should adjust their dosage accordingly. Typically, the more overweight one is, the better they can tolerate thermogenic substances; however, this must be assessed individually. Because several thermogenic formulas exist, look for products that come from reliable manufacturers. Ephedra-based thermogenic combinations can be very effective weight loss tools and, if used judiciously, can provide a safe and efficient way to burn fat stores and to maintain an ideal weight.

CHAPTER 6

SUGAR, MUSCLE AND FAT

One of the most difficult obstacles to effective and permanent weight loss is the persistent feeling of unsatisfied hunger. Hunger pains are meant to signal an urgent metabolic need for food, however, as we've discussed, we are beginning to understand that brain chemistry can greatly influence appetite. Ideally, if our nutritional requirements are being met, we should not feel hungry. For many of us, this is simply not the case. Binging on carbohydrates affects a great number of people who consistently crave foods that raise blood sugar.

Using artificial sweeteners like aspartame or saccharine in an attempt to cut back on calories is not recommended. Current data suggests that these substances may not only pose significant health risks, they often confuse the body and create more problems. Artificial sweeteners are not the panacea they are assumed to be—as is the case with so many chemically derived substances. Luckily, nature has provided us with some excellent noncaloric sweeteners.

OUR OBSESSION WITH SUGAR

Ralph Nader once said, "If God meant us to eat sugar, he wouldn't have invented dentists." The average American eats over 125 pounds of white sugar every year. It has ben estimated that sugar makes up 25 percent of our daily caloric intake, with soda pop supplying the majority of our sugar ingestion. Desserts and sugar-laden snacks continually tempt us, resulting in an escalated taste for sweets. The amount of sugar we consume as a country has a profound effects on both our physical and mental well-being. Sugar is a powerful substance which can have drug-like effects and is considered addictive by some nutritional experts. William Duffy, author of *Sugar Blues*, states, "The difference between sugar addiction and narcotic addition is largely one of degree."

In excess, sugar can be toxic, Sufficient amounts of B-vitamins are actually required to metabolize and detoxify sugar in our bodies. When the body experiences a sugar overload, the assimilation of nutrients from other foods can be inhibited. In other words, our bodies were not designed to cope with the enormous quantity of sugar we routinely ingest. Eating too much sugar can generate a type of nutrient malnutrition, not to mention its contribution to obesity, diabetes, hyperactivity, etc. etc. Sugar can also predispose the body to yeast infections, aggravate some types of arthritis and asthma, cause tooth decay and may even elevate blood lipid levels.

Eating excess sugar can also contribute to amino acid depletion, which has been linked with depression and other mood disorders. To make matters worse, eating too much sugar can actually compromise our immune systems by lowering white blood cells counts. This makes us more susceptible to colds and other infections. Sugar consumption has also been linked to PMS, osteoporosis and coronary heart disease.

Why Do We Crave Sweets?

Considering the sobering effects of a high sugar diet, why to we eat so much of it? One reason is that sugar gives us a quick infusion of energy. It can also help to raise the level of certain brain neurotransmitters which temporality may elevate our mood. Sugar cravings stem from a complex mix of physiological and psychological components. Even the most brilliant scientists fail to totally comprehend this intriguing chemical dependence which, for the most part, hurts our overall health.

What we do know is that when sugary foods are consumed, the pancreas must secrete insulin, a hormone which serves to bring blood glucose levels down. This allows sugar to enter our cells where it is either burned off or stored. The constant up and down of blood sugar levels can become exaggerated in some individuals and cause all kinds of health problems. Have you ever been around someone who is prone to sudden mood swings characterized by violent verbal attacks or irritability? This type of volatile behavior is typical of some people who crave sugar, eat it and then experience sugar highs and lows. Erratic mood swings can be linked to dramatic drops in blood sugar levels.

Artificial Sweeteners: Cause for Worry

Among some of the most troubling food additives that we routinely ingest are artificial sweeteners, also referred to as non-nutritive sweeteners. Having received the FDA stamp of approval, they are liberally ingested with little thought as to what their actual health risks may be. Andrew Weil, M.D., in his book *Natural Health Natural Medicine,* writes:

> More worrisome than preservatives are artificial sweeteners. Saccharin, a known carcinogen, should be avoided. Cyclamates, banned some years ago for suspected carcinogenicity, are not being reconsidered for use in food. They taste better than saccharin but cause diarrhea in some people. Avoid them too. Recently, aspartame (NutraSweet) has become enormously popular. The manufacturer portrays it as a gift from nature, but, although the two component amino acids occur in nature, aspartame itself does not. Like all artificial sweeteners, aspartame has a peculiar taste. Because I have seen a number of patients, mostly women, who report

headaches from this substance, I don't regard it as free from toxicity. Women also find that aspartame aggravates, PMS (premenstrual syndrome). I think you are better off using moderate amounts of sugar than consuming any artificial sweeteners on a regular basis. A natural sweetener that may cause some people problems is sorbitol, originally derived from the berries of the mountain ash tree. Sorbitol tastes sweet but is not easily absorbed from the gastrointestinal tract and is not easily metabolized. It is a common ingredient of sugarless chewing gums and candies. If you eat a lot of it, you will probably get diarrhea. People with irritable bowel syndrome or ulcerative colitis should avoid sorbitol.

Ann Louise Gittleman, in her book *Super Nutrition for Women,* writes:

> In 1977 a Canadian study indicated that when pregnant rats were fed large doses of saccharin, their male offspring developed bladder cancer. As a result, the Canadians banned saccharin and the U.S. Congress ordered warning labels on all saccharin products like Sweet 'N Low. In 1978 the National Academy of Sciences evaluated the evidence and concluded that saccharin was primarily a promoter of other cancer-causing agents—a cocarcinogen. In the meantime, G.D. Searle developed aspartame, a combination of two amino acids and methanol (wood alcohol) . . . Few long-term studies on the effects of aspartame have been done. However, reports to the FDA and the Center for Disease Control indicate that, as more people consume the substitute in large quantities, health may be affected. In some circumstances, individuals may be getting high levels of methanol; for example, it is estimated that on a hot day after exercise, an individual drinking three 12-ounce cans of diet cola could easily consume as much as eight times the Environmental Protection Agency's recommended limit for methanol consumption. The most common complaints are dizziness, disorientation, tunnel vision, ear buzzing, loss of equilibrium, numbing of hands and feet,

inflammation of the pancreas, high blood pressure, eye hemorrhages and seizures. Artificial sweeteners can stimulate hunger or cause additive allergies, just as sugar does. In other words, we get the disadvantages of sugar, along with the proven or suspected disadvantages of artificial sweeteners.

While thousands of Americans continue to consume aspartame in unprecedented amounts, controversy surrounding its safety lingers. Dr. Richard Wurtman of the Massachusetts Institute of Technology (MIT) has reported that abnormal concentrations of neurotransmitters developed when he fed laboratory animals large doses of aspartame. He believes that the phenylalanine content of the sweetener actually manipulates and alters certain brain chemicals which could initiate behavioral changes and even seizures. He also purports that while small quantities of aspartame may be safe, the cumulative effects of the compound—particularly if consumed with high-carbohydrate, low-protein snacks—could be serious.[51] In spite of serious concerns, saccharine and aspartame packets sit in restaurant sugar bowls all over our country.

The FDA and Current Noncaloric Sweeteners

While white sugar, turbinado, fructose, honey and corn syrup all qualify as natural sweeteners, none of these are calorie-free nor can they be used by people who suffer from blood sugar disorders. They encourage weight gain, promote tooth decay, raise blood sugar quickly, and can also predispose certain individuals to yeast infections. These sugars can also contribute to indigestion, bowel disorders and hyperactivity or ADD in children.

Pharmaceutical sweeteners like saccharin and aspartame qualify as calorie-free but come with significant limitations and health risks. Saccharin has been labeled with a warning that it causes the development of cancer in laboratory animals, but it is still available for purchase. Aspartame has been marketed as a safe substance for the general public, except for those few individuals who suffer from PKU (phenylketonuria). Most consumers assume that aspartame is a perfectly benign compound and use it liberally. It is, in fact, comprised of phenylalanine, aspartic acid, and methanol. As previously mentioned, various side effects have been associated with the ingestion of aspartame and include migraines, memory loss, slurred speech, dizziness, stomach pain, and even seizures.

In addition, because aspartame contains chemicals which affect brain cell function, significant questions have been raised concerning its link to increased incidence of brain tumors.[52] Acesulfame K, another artificial sweetener on the market, has also been linked to cancer by the Center for Science. Despite the protest of various organizations and health professionals, these pharmaceutical sweeteners have been approved by the FDA and are recognized as safe.

STEVIA

Stevia is an herb with incredible sweetening power. Its ability to sweeten is rated between 70 to 400 times that of white sugar. Typically, it has a mild licorice-like taste and is completely natural in its biochemical profile. What makes stevia so intriguing is that unlike other natural sweetening agents, its is completely calorie-free, never initiates a rise in blood sugar and does not provide food for microorganisms like bacterias and yeasts.

Stevia may well be the most remarkable sweetener in the world and yet its recognition in this country remains relatively low. Consider the extraordinary attributes of the stevia plant and its extracts.

- 50 to 400 times sweeter than white sugar
- does not adversely effect blood sugar levels
- inhibits formation of cavities and plaque
- no artificial ingredients
- diabetic-safe
- calorie free
- nontoxic
- used in baking

For anyone who suffers from diabetes, hypoglycemia, high blood pressure, obesity or chronic yeast infections, stevia is the ideal sweetener. It has all the benefits of artificial sweeteners and none of the drawbacks. Stevia can be added to a variety of foods to make them sweet without adding calories or impacting the pancreas or adrenal glands. It can also help to satisfy carbohydrate cravings without interfering with blood sugar levels or adding extra pounds.

Using stevia to create treats for children is an excellent way to avoid weight gain, tooth decay and possible hyperactivity. While they may take some getting used to initially, stevia products are becoming easier to measure and are better tasting.

Stevia and Blood Sugar Levels

Clinical tests combined with consumer results indicate that stevia can actually help to normalize blood sugar. For this reason, the herb and its extracts are recommended in some countries as an actual medicine for people suffering from diabetes or hypoglycemia. Recent studies have indicated that stevia can increase glucose tolerance while decreasing blood sugar levels.

Paraguayan natives have traditionally used stevia tea to regulate blood sugar. Stevia decoctions for diabetes are common and are usually prepared by boiling or steeping the leaves in water.[53] It is thought that while disturbed blood sugar levels respond to stevia therapy, normal levels remain unaffected. Scientific studies are certainly warranted.

Stevia and Weight Loss

Stevia is an ideal dietary supplement for anyone who wants to lose or maintain weight. Because it contains no calories, it can satisfy cravings for sweets without adding extra pounds. It is also thought that using stevia may decrease the desire to eat fatty foods. Appetite control is another factor affected by stevia supplementation. Some people have found that their hunger decreases if they take stevia drops fifteen to twenty minutes before a meal. While scientific studies are lacking in this area, it is presumed that the glycosides in stevia help to reset the appestat mechanism found in the brain, thereby promoting a feeling of satiety or satisfaction.

Much of our nation's obesity epidemic is due to the over consumption of sugar-containing foods. (And most sugary snacks are loaded with fat, which compounds the problem.) When a sugar craving hits, anything will usually do. Using stevia to sweeten snacks and beverages can result in making weight management much easier.

Safety: The FDA has not given stevia the "generally recognized as safe" label; however, the herbal compound has been used for hundreds of years without any recorded side effects. Japanese studies have found that the sweetener consistently yields a non-toxic status, even after extensive toxicity trials. Stevia has been used for years in Japan with the approval of Japanese control agencies. In Paraguay, the herb has enjoyed hundreds of years of consumption with no reports of detrimental side effects. No anomalies have ever been observed in cell, enzyme, chromosomal or other significant physiological parameters during toxicity tests. The herb has not been associated with any form of cancer or birth defects. Stevia consumption in Japan was approximated at 170 metric tons in 1987 with no cases of documented side effects.[54]

Scientific Toxicology Studies

Comprehensive and tedious clinical studies in Japan have more than established the fact that stevia can be taken safely. One study used over 450 rats who were fed stevia for up to two years with doses many times greater than human consumption. No changes were observed in organ weights, blood biochemistry, growth, appearance or cellular function.[55] The Japanese have found no indication that stevia affects fertility or unborn children and have never linked it to cancer or other cellular mutations. (*Note:* Diabetics and individuals with other medical conditions should always consult their physician before using this or any other dietary supplement. They should also never alter or stop their medication unless advised to do so by their physician.)

Forms of Stevia

Stevia has traditionally been used in either a powder or a raw liquid form. Powdered forms can either be crude and green or fine and white; they come in bulk or in tea bags. White stevia powder is the most common type and usually has more sweetening power than other forms. Countries like Japan use a filler substance along with the powder to give it more substance and make it easier to package. Powdered forms can be somewhat difficult to measure, although they are considered quite practical. Liquid formulas are often added to other compounds to counteract bitterness. New concentrated liquid varieties are also available, as are alcohol-based stevia extracts. Fresh leaves can be chewed but they are not practical for sweetening other foods. Stevia tablets are available for those who want to use the herb as a therapeutic rather than sweetening agent. Ground stevia can be sprinkled over cereals, salads, and other ready-to-serve foods. (*Note:* Stevia powders can vary in their sweetening strength which is determined to a great degree by the refining process and the plant quality.)

MUSCLE VS. FAT

In this section the link between lean muscle, fat and blood sugar will be addressed. Understanding the biochemical mechanisms related to fat burning in muscle mass and its relationship to blood sugar is vitally important to weight control.

When fatty tissue is present, muscle mass is usually decreased. Muscles that are out of shape lose their ability to respond to insulin. Consequently, blood sugar levels are adversely affected. The goal of any good weight-loss strategy should be the promotion of lean muscle mass because it burns off more calories and keeps insulin secretion in check. Because glucose intolerance is frequently found in overweight people, supplements that help stabilize blood sugar and prompt the formation of lean muscle tissue are crucial. It's no coincidence that individuals who battle the bulge are frequently diabetic or hypoglycemic. One study found that women who carry excess fat in their upper bodies are eight times ore likely to develop diabetes than other women.[56]

An excessive insulin response can trigger ravenous hunger which usually results in a glut of carbohydrate consumption and fat storage. Interestingly, high levels of insulin make it easier for food, regardless of its makeup, to convert to fat stores rather than to energy or heat. Several natural compounds help to normalize insulin secretion and sugar utilization on a cellular level, thereby preventing abnormal carbohydrate eating binges.

Chromium Picolinate or GTF Chromium

Chromium is a mineral that inhibits sugar cravings by helping to stabilize the metabolism of simple sugars or carbohydrates. More often than not, our appestat center reacts to blood sugar levels. Chromium has the ability to boost the function of insulin which enables sugar to leave the bloodstream and enter cells. When sugar passes through cell membranes our desire to eat should lessen. The way in which we metabolize sugars is critical to how we feel, both mentally and physically. False hunger pains or unusual cravings for sweets are intrinsically linked to brain chemistry and glucose levels. Chromium can help to keep our appestats in control by helping us to avoid the kind of binge eating that puts on the pounds. A 1994 study found that chromium directly affects the insulin activity of brain cells, significantly impacting the hypothalamus which is profoundly involved in the regulation of appetite and burning of fat.

Scientific evidence supports the fact that chromium can help to normalize blood sugar and discourage storage of fat.

Safety Issues: The range in which chromium is therapeutically effective is quite narrow. An excess or overdose of chromium can actually inhibit rather than enhance insulin activity. If you are taking any medications for diabetes or high cholesterol, check with your doctor before taking chromium supplements. No toxicity has been observed in oral sources of chromium at this writing.

Glucomannan (*Amorphophallus konjak*)

Glucomannan is a unique herb which provides dietary fiber with no calories. It promotes bowel elimination, absorbs intestinal toxins and can help normalize blood sugar. In addition, when taken before meals this herb can help produce a feeling of fullness which suppresses the appetite. As a diet aid, it can expand to about fifty times its original volume when combined with water. Glucomannan is currently being used in weight reduction formulas to suppress carbohydrate cravings. When combined with lecithin, it is thought to help prevent cardiovascular disease. In an experimental double-blind study involving twenty obese subjects, those who took one gram of glucomannan one hour prior to each meal without altering their eating or exercise habits experienced a significant mean weight loss with no side effects whatsoever.[57]

Safety Issues: This herb is considered nontoxic, but anyone with any blood sugar-related disease should check with their physician before using glucomannan.

Gymnema (*Gymnema sylvestre*)

Gymnema leaves have the remarkable ability to block out certain taste sensations, especially sweetness. The herb is extremely popular in Japan and is included in diabetic, hypoglycemic and weight-loss formulas. Modern research has found the gymnemic acid, the active ingredient of the herb, blocks sugar absorption into the body.[58] A clinical study published in 1986 suggests that extract of gymnema can significantly enhance liver and pancreatic function.[59]

Safety Issues: Diabetics should check with their physician before using this herb.

L-Glutamine

Some recent studies have found that using glutamine can reduce the desire for sugary foods as well as alcohol cravings.[60] In addition, glutamine helps to build and maintain muscle tissue, a fact which makes it a favorite supplement for body builders and people wishing to increasing lean muscle mass. Using between 200 mg and one gram of glutamine has demonstrated this effect. Take glutamine thirty minutes before meals to lessen the desire for carbohydrates.

Safety Issues: Glutamine should not be taken by people with liver or kidney disease, anyone with Rey's syndrome, or individuals with conditions related to ammonia build up in the blood.

L-Carnitine

Carnitine cannot in the strictest chemical sense be called an amino acid, although it is usually listed with other amino acids. It is an important addition to thermogenic formulas in that it assists in the transport of long-chain fatty acids which are burned for energy. In this way, carnitine enhances the consumption of fat as a source of fuel. It plays a major role in mobilizing fatty deposits found in the tissues of overweight individuals and helps to remove ketones (fat waste products) from the bloodstream. This particular action helps to discourage fatty buildup in organs like the heart and liver and in skeletal muscle. Such buildup occurs in conditions which are often related to diseases like diabetes, heart disease and obesity. As mentioned earlier, lean muscle mass burns calories and carnitine can contribute to improved muscle strength. In addition, carnitine actually reduces certain triglycerides in the blood and elevates HDL cholesterol (the good kind).[61] Consider the following quote:

> The primary function of carnitine in the body is to regulate fat oxidation. Fats are produced in the body as well as being derived from the diet, and it is when the body's fat-regulating mechanisms don't get the nutrition they need to function properly that we have the onset of major biochemical problems. Carnitine is the key balancing nutrient in this case.[62]

L-carnitine is the preferred form of this amino acid. Adding L-methionine, another amino acid, is thought to improve the effectiveness of carnitine. Taking between 50 to 300 mg of carnitine per day is recommended.

Safety Issues: Carnitine should not be used by anyone with kidney disorders. Some individuals have reported some gastrointestinal side effects from usage.

CHAPTER 7

PROPER DIGESTION AND ELIMINATION FOR WEIGHT CONTROL

It is no secret that great numbers of Americans have trouble digesting the food they so eagerly pop into their mouths. Poor digestion coupled with inadequate elimination sets the body up for inevitable weight gain. Moreover, impaired food assimilation and the improper expulsion of waste material makes weight loss much more difficult to achieve. When we fail to assimilate nutrients efficiently, we may develop a condition called malabsorption. This condition causes cravings, abnormal appetites and binging which indicate that the body's homeostatic balances are out of whack and which also lead to weight gain.

We are all aware of the fact that most of us eat much more food than our body should be required to process. Digestive enzymes can help us to better digest and assimilate food, thereby resulting in decreased food intake. If we were eating enough raw, fresh foods, we may not be enzymatically deficient. It is the cooked or processed foods which contain no enzymes.

DIGESTIVE ENZYMES

Taking a good digestive enzyme supplement can help to boost digestion which contributes to good calorie burning. Our diets often lack important compounds that promote nutrient assimilation and the production of energy. Our systems become sluggish, making us susceptible to weight gain. Supplementing with enzymes helps to jump start our digestive processes and makes it easier to efficiently burn fuel rather than store it as fat.

Pancreatin

Using pancreatin supplementation can help to boost enzyme function. Clinical tests using laboratory animals resulted in a marked decrease in food consumption and a significant loss of body weight.[63]

Papain

Derived from papaya fruit, this enzyme helps to breakdown protein and gluten. A high-protein diet is one of the reasons people suffer from so many gastrointestinal disorders. Undigested protein has been linked to autoimmune diseases and other ailments which have no known cause.

Bromelain

The pineapple plant supplies this enzyme which breaks down protein and acts as a natural anti-inflammatory agent. It works best when used in conjunction with pancreatin

THE COLON CONNECTION

The connection between obesity and the colon is a facet of weight management that should not be overlooked. It is believed that for the mechanisms of weight loss to operate at maximum efficiency, the proper elimination of waste from the body must be ensured. Unfortunately, most of us eat diets that have a tendency to promote rather than prevent constipation. In the case of thermogenics, the connection is very important because of the possible constipating effect of thermogenic compounds.

The notion of autointoxication may also play a role in weight control. When the bowel is sluggish, toxins can be reabsorbed and nutrients malabsorbed. As a result, the body's appestat can become stimulated, creating abnormal hunger and food cravings. Eating a diet high in fiber or taking a good fiber supplement can prevent constipation. In addition herbal formulas containing cascara sagrada can be excellent and mild purgatives.

Regularity and Weight Control

Americans spend more on laxatives than any other country in the world. Last year laxative sales were conservatively placed at $350 million, a sad commentary on the deplorable state of colon health. The fact that weight reduction can be significantly inhibited by chronic constipation must be considered when choosing an effectual way to lose and keep off weight. For the mechanisms of weight loss to operate at maximum efficiency, the proper elimination of waste from the body must be insured.

The homeostatic mechanisms of the body should keep the bloodstream free from impurities, but when the colon is not operating as it should, toxins can be reabsorbed. Keep in mind that getting rid of waste material and toxic substances must take place efficiently right down to the cellular level. For all these reasons, fiber can play an invaluable role in weight management.

FIBER AND WEIGHT CONTROL

While most of us know how important it is to reduce the amount of fat we consume, many of us remain oblivious to the profound role that fiber plays in helping to keep our arteries clear, preventing obesity and expediting toxins from the bowel. Ideally, a decrease in dietary fats combined with an increase in fiber and exercise comprise the winning prescription for preventing not only obesity but also a whole host of other diseases.

Fiber is an important indigestible plant material found in fruits, grains and vegetables. Cultures that routinely eat high fiber diets have a very low incidence of obesity. Unquestionably, these people do not count calories to maintain an ideal weight. High-fiber diets expedite the excretion of fat in the stool, improve glucose tolerance and help to provide a feeling of fullness in the stomach. In this way the right kind of fiber can act as an appetite suppressant.

In the March 1984 edition of the *Saturday Evening Post,* Dr. Cory SerVas reported that fiber reduces the absorption of fat and by drawing water into the intestinal system, creates a sensation of fullness with less caloric intake. Some studies have shown that when nutritious, high fiber diets are consumed, food cravings diminish. Dietary fiber also helps to guard against constipation by increasing the volume and fluid content of the stool. In so doing, bowel congestion is alleviated and transit time is decreased.

It is worth mentioning that eating a diet high in fiber is believed to help remove excess estrogen in women. Of interest is the fact that the more fat a woman carries, the more estrogen she produces and the hungrier she feels. The role of fiber in promoting and maintaining regularity cannot be overemphasized. Dietary fiber can prevent and treat obesity by:

- slowing the eating process by increasing required chewing
- increasing the excretion of fat in the feces
- improving digestive hormone secretion and digestion
- improving glucose tolerance
- inducing a feeling of fullness
- stimulating the release of intestinal hormones that reduce food intake[64]

Psyllium

Called the "mother of herbs" in Anglo-Saxon literature, psyllium provides an excellent source of dietary fiber. Its tiny seeds are coated with mucilage, a gelatinous substance that swells when it comes in contact with moisture. For this reason psyllium is referred to as a *hemicellulose,* a substance which stimulates the colon without irritating intestinal tissue. Psyllium also helps to lubricate and heal the intestinal tract. It is an excellent bulking agent that gently promotes regularity. The combination of increased fluid and fiber can significantly boost the process of weight loss. In his book *The Scientific Validation of Herbal Medicine,* Daniel Mowrey states:

> In Italy, a study on the effects of [psyllium] in a reducing diet for women who averaged about 60 percent overweight resulted in weight loss greater than that obtained by the diet alone . . . The effects of [psyllium] on weight loss was dramatic. In summary, it appears that [psyllium] produces weight loss by limiting caloric intake, due to its appetite-satiating effect, and by reduced intestinal absorption of lipids.

Fiber Supplements: A Dieter's Best Friend

Because most of us have good intentions but rarely meet our optimal dietary goals, fiber supplementation is recommended. Ideally we should be eating enough fibery foods in the form of fruits, vegetables and whole grains. Realistically, we usually fall short, no matter how dedicated we might be. If we have any type of glucose impairment disorder like diabetes, we may not be able to eat the amount of fruit recommended. We may never develop a taste for whole grain cereals or may be guilty of consistent meal skipping. If we are allergic to grains like wheat, obtaining enough fiber could be significantly more difficult.

Finding a high quality fiber supplement is highly recommended. If you're going to purchase a fiber supplement, make sure that it is a vegetable based formula. The advantages of taking a fiber supplement are many:

- It's an easy way to fortify your diet with fiber two to three times a day if desired.
- Vegetable fibers that have been ground to powders can make the fiber source more digestible.

- Fiber formulas can contain sources of fiber as well as other nutrients or herbs that we normally don't consume—rice bran, guar gum, pectin, gum acacia, locust bean gum, psyllium and aloe vera.
- Fiber supplements sometimes contain a variety of fiber sources which are preferable to just one fiber food. Different types of fiber initiate different physiological responses in the body.
- Fiber supplements can be taken anywhere.
- Taking a fiber supplement on a daily basis helps to lower cholesterol levels, speed transit time, prevent constipation and contribute to weight management.

Types of Fiber Supplements

- Bran fiber: Poor solubility with good water holding properties
- Psyllium: Colorless transparent mucilage forms around the insoluble seed
- Gums: Forms a homogenous adhesive gelatinous mass to expedite colonic waste
- Methyl cellulose: Slowly soluble and creates a viscous, colloid solution
- Ispaghula husk: Swells rapidly to form a still mucilage

Any of these fiber supplements can be enhanced by adding:

- Herbs such as aloe vera, cascara sagrada, rhubarb, slippery elm or acacia (each of these herbs exerts a toning or healing effect on the mucous membranes of the colon).
- Calcium, which can help to protect the colon from the development of malignancies.
- GTF chromium, which increases insulin utilization and when taken with fiber contributes to normalizing blood sugar levels which affects food cravings and fat storage.
- Hitamins and minerals: B-vitamins, biotin, vitamin E, ascorbic acid and zinc only improve the nutritive value of the fiber mix.

Fiber supplements are usually available in powder form and are designed to mix with a liquid. They are typically blended into juices, hot cereals, casseroles, dressings, and gravies. if you find them difficult to take in drink form, think of creative ways to sneak them into moist food like soups, stews, or batters (pancakes, waffles, cookies, cakes, etc.). Experience has proven that if you add fiber supplements to your diet, they work better if you rotate them. Popular and effective supplements include gum acacia, pectin, guar gum, oat fiber, psyllium seed, apple pectin, agar and flaxseed. For optimal results, make sure you get adequate amounts of the fiber preparations.

Remember that you need to take fiber supplement for at least three months before you will begin to see consistent physiological benefits. Begin by adding fiber slowly to your diet and try not to overdose on just one type of fiber. Fiber formulas that include a variety of fiber or a mix of vitamins, herbs or minerals are especially good. Take your fiber supplement thirty minutes before you eat to help create satiety and drink plenty of water—at least eight glasses a day.

HERBS THAT PROMOTE ELIMINATION

Cascara Sagrada (*Rhamnus purshiana*)

Cascara sagrada is an excellent herbal purgative and digestive tonic. North American Indians traditionally used this botanical as a natural laxative and referred to it as "sacred bark." Cascara sagrada promotes regularity without becoming habit forming. It is rich in hormone-like oils which initiate peristaltic action in the intestinal tract. The herb has a remarkable toning action on the bowel and can restore normal function. It also helps to detoxify liver cells which act to filter out waste products harmful to the body.

Senna (*Cassia acutifolia*)

Traditionally found along the banks of the Nile in Egypt and Sudan, senna leaves and pods were used in ancient Arabic medicine as safe and effective laxatives. Senna acts as a remarkable stimulant to the intestinal tract tissue. Because it has a strong laxative effect, senna is conducive to colon cleansing. Taking ginger in combination with senna helps to prevent bowel cramping that may occur with any purgative botanical. The compounds in senna are absorbed in the small intestine and act on the nerves of the colon to simulate peristaltic action.

Buckthorn (*Rhamnus frangula*)

According to the writings of the Greek physician Galen, buckthorn was used medicinally as early as the second century A.D. Buckthorn tea has long been a favorite herbal remedy for constipation. It is particularly valuable for its ability to promote bowel movements without the typical cramping usually associated with laxatives. Like cascara sagrada, buckthorn can be used indefinitely without the development of a dependence on the substance.

The natural laxative action of herbs that promote elimination should be combined with carminative herbs such as ginger, peppermint and fennel. Carminative herbs serve to stimulate enzyme production which can prevent intestinal discomfort. The key to effective cleansing is to supplement any colon purge with herbs designed to nutritionally support the digestive system.

LIVER SUPPORT FOR WEIGHT LOSS

Boosting liver function is necessary in virtually all weight loss programs but is often neglected. The liver is the primary organ involved in purifying the blood of impurities and in the metabolism of fat. Liver support must be an integral part of any effective weight reduction strategy. Certain herbs and other compounds can hasten the removal of fat from the liver. Liver function is disturbed in a large percentage of overweight individuals.[65]

Research has discovered that a significant number of overweight individuals also suffer from impaired liver function. One of the liver's primary functions is to metabolize fats, a function intrinsically linked to weight control. Certain natural compounds enhance and support the liver's ability to break down lipids. For example, herbs which stimulate bile flow from the gall bladder to the liver help to facilitate this function and other natural agents can help to boost the removal of fats from the liver. Oregon grape root, dandelion and milk thistle help to improve liver function and so play an integral part in weight loss. The liver also plays a role in maintaining stable blood sugar levels, a biofunction which is profoundly connected to hunger and weight management.

Attractylodes macrocephala Extract

It is vitally important to keep fluids moving out of the body during the course of any weight loss program. Burning fat causes the creation of waste products which must be eliminated through both the bowels and the kidneys. Flushing body tissues with pure water, combined with the assistance of certain diuretic herbs, helps to keep fat by-products from building up.

Attractylodes macrocephala is a Chinese herb that has the ability to facilitate the elimination of tissue fluids by reducing levels of sodium. As we all know, sodium promotes fluid retention and can raise blood pressure under certain circumstances. Other herbs which have natural diuretic actions and help to prevent water retention are uva ursi, buchu, shave grass, cornsilk, cranberry, parsley, hydrangea, watermelon seed, and juniper berries.

CHAPTER 8

OTHER INGREDIENTS IN WEIGHT-LOSS FORMULAS

N atural weight loss formulas often contain a wide variety of strange sounding herbs and compounds. The selection of these substances is usually based on the individual contribution of each herb, mineral or other supplement. The following is a list of secondary ingredients you may observe on the labels of weight loss products and their primary function.

Capsicum

Capsicum or cayenne pepper has a stimulatory effect on the body and can contribute to the creation of heat which occurs when energy is expended or wasted. It also works as an overall catalyst which serves to enhance the actions of other compounds with which it is combined.

Kelp and Bladderwrack

Some formulas include kelp to help stimulate the thyroid gland. This increases our physiological ability to burn fat when we exercise. Thyroid function determines, to a great degree, our metabolic rates. 225 mg per day of kelp is recommended.

Vanadium

Considered a trace mineral, vanadium helps to transport glycogen (stored sugar) to muscle tissue where it can be used to promote lean muscle mass or is burned for energy.

Inositol

Involved in glucose metabolism, this compound may augment weight loss and lower cholesterol levels. It is used in the metabolism of fats. The recommended dosage is 500 to 1500 mg per day.

Lecithin

Considered a fat emulsifier, lecithin contains choline which is involved in the transport of fats and cholesterol in the body. 1000 mg per day is the recommended dosage.

Gaba

Gaba helps to suppress food cravings and contributes to mood elevation.

Vitamin B6 (Pyridoxine)

Vitamin B6 serves as an essential coenzyme for normal amino acid metabolism. It is also vital to properly metabolize dietary fats, carbohydrates and proteins. 100 mg per day is recommended.

Vitamin C

Clinical trials have suggested that vitamin C may reduce obesity by increasing the amount of energy consumed in the cells. It achieves this affect by influencing cellular sodium pump activity. Two clinical trials both involving double blind studies found that using one gram or more of ascorbic acid daily led to significant weight loss without any calorie restriction.[66]

Potassium Citrate

Potassium citrate is an easily absorbable form of potassium which is stored almost exclusively in lean tissue. It controls muscle contractibility and nerve transmission and is essential to maintain normal blood pressure.

Borage Oil and Bitter Orange Oil

These are sometimes added to weight loss formulas as appetite suppressants which also contain essential fatty acids which help to promote fat burning.

It is important to continually supply the body with a full array of vitamins and minerals at all times, but during weight loss it is particularly relevant. Using protein and vitamin shakes coupled with supplemental digestive enzymes and phytonutrients helps to provide human tissue with added nutrition. Vitamins A, B1, B3, B6, B12, C, E, GABA and folic acid, combined with zinc, potassium, calcium/magnesium, manganese, selenium, boron and phosphate, are recommended.

CHAPTER 9

A WORD ON DIETING

Unfortunately, attempting to initiate weight loss by dieting often results in compromised health and diminished self esteem. Why do 97 percent of all diets ultimately fail? Why are 33 billion dollars spent on weight loss programs that don't work, and why are we more overweight now than we've ever been before? The average American has gained eight pounds over the last ten years. Statistics tell us that two out of three people who go on a diet regain the weight in one year or less. Ninety-seven percent will regain the weight in five years. Obesity in children has more than doubled since the 1950s and the average weights for both males and females continue to increase.

Human physiology responds to dieting the same way it does to the potential threat of starvation—it turns its engines down. Consequently, the body burns less fuel and stores it much more readily. In this way the very act of dieting can serve as a self-defeating exercise. It seems obvious that dieting has not solved the problem of weight gain but what it has done is create havoc with human metabolic processes. More than a few people have lived through the vicious cycle of weight loss followed by weight gain only to go on yet another diet.

In reality, there is no diet that can cure obesity and there never will be. The business of losing weight has become more of a recurring syndrome rather than a health-promoting activity.

Health is frequently sacrificed in exchange for burning fat, a fact that only serves to compound weight problems and compromise vitality. Ironically, calorie restriction, the basis of dieting, only serves to force the body to protect itself against the threat of a diminished supply of fuel. This protective mode inhibits the body's ability to release and burn fat. In addition, an increased production of enzymes known as lipoprotein lipase (LPL) assists fat cells in scavenging for any lipids present in the blood stream. Drastic weight reduction diets can put this enzyme into over-drive. Months after dieting is stopped, this enzyme can remain abnormally active, making it more difficult to return to eating normal quantities of food without gaining weight.

Because the body is engineered toward self preservation, when it is threatened through starvation diets, fat is conserved for future energy reserves. As a result of this nutrient hoarding, hunger is produced, more eating results, and the malicious cycle continues.

STANDARD MEDICAL TREATMENTS FOR OBESITY:

Obesity is extremely difficult to treat successfully. Most physicians suggest a diet that will usually lower caloric intake to 1500 calories per day combined with fifteen to twenty minutes of aerobic exercise for at least three to four times weekly. Gradual weight loss is recommended (1/2 pound to one pound per week). Diets are usually designed to take advantage of all five food groups recommended for good health.

Anti-obesity drugs such as nonamphetamine appetite suppressants are sometimes prescribed by physicians; however, their use is discouraged due to their side effects. Drugs which are designed to increase the body's energy requirements are currently being tested. Antidepressant drugs such as Prozac are also being currently investigated for their possible role in weight loss.

Many nonamphetamine appetite suppressant drugs have side effects similar to those of amphetamines. Some of the side effects are nervousness, restlessness, sleeplessness, palpitations, high blood pressure, drowsiness, dizziness, headache, tremors and over stimulation. (*Warning:* The drug dimitrophinol, which is prescribed by some physicians for weight loss, may cause cataracts.)

Wiring the teeth together to prohibit eating is another possible medical treatment for obesity. The treatment is uncomfortable and while it may produce results, they are usually temporary and have nothing to do with eating habit modification. In addition, wiring the jaw may promote tooth decay and mouth infections.

Surgical Options

Liposuction is a procedure that involves making an incision through which a tube is placed to suck out fat cells. The procedure is extremely traumatic to surrounding tissue and causes a considerable amount of bruising and pain. There is the possibility of developing a blood clot from this procedure, a situation which could be life-threatening.

A colectomy is a type of bypass surgery that reduces the area of intestine through which food can be absorbed. It can also decrease appetite. This is considered a major surgical procedure and carries with it the risk of serious complications or death. The proper assimilation of vitamins and minerals is also impaired. The use of this particular surgery has declined due to its adverse effects.

Stomach stapling reduces the size of the stomach, therefore limiting the amount of food which can be ingested at one time. This is a major surgical procedure which carries with it serious complications or the risk of death. In some instances the staples do not hold and the surgery has to be repeated. Eating disturbances such as involuntary regurgitation can result from this procedure.

A high percentage of people who use drastic surgical procedures to lose weight do eventually gain it back. The success rate of standard medical treatments for obesity is very poor and the treatments often prove frustrating for both patient and doctor. Drugs and drastic surgical procedures also come with a number of negative side effects.

ADDITIONAL WEIGHT LOSS TIPS

- Exercise regularly. Exercise is considered by far the best method to control weight. Begin slowly. Take a ten to fifteen minute walk every day and then slowly increase your distance and your pace. Light exercise right after eating is recommended to help burn calories that have just been consumed.
- Don't become constipated. Drink six to eight glasses of water per day.
- Don't chew gum. Chewing gum can activate the flow of gastric juices and make you feel like eating.
- Eat only when you are truly hungry. Thirst can often be mistaken for hunger so drink when you feel the urge to eat.
- Avoid eating when you are anxious, bored or frustrated. Find something else to do when you feel inclined to eat under these circumstances.
- Don't eat while reading or watching T.V. As fun as this might be, it promotes inactivity and weight gain. If you have to eat during these activities, munch on raw veggies. Television watching, video games, etc. have greatly decreased the amount of physical activity children pursue. These sedentary activities have been strongly linked to obesity.
- Avoid nibbling after the meal is over. Mothers are particularly susceptible to this. While they may eat sensibly during the meal, picking at leftovers while putting dishes away can significantly contribute to weight gain.
- Try not to use food as a reward.

- Keep all high-calorie foods on high shelves or in the back of the refrigerator. Low-cal foods should be easily accessible.
- Eating too fast or improper chewing can result in the overconsumption of calories during a certain period of time. Eating a diet that is high in fiber can automatically increase chewing time and slow the eating process. People who eat too fast can often become hungry again soon after eating. Listen to calm, soothing music while you eat and chew slowly.
- Don't eat when you are depressed, lonely or angry.
- Avoid fad diets which can make your body feel as if its starving and actually lower your metabolism which slows the burning of fat stores.
- Do not use diuretics or laxative to induce weight loss. These can be potentially hazardous to your health and result in temporary weight loss only.
- Join a support group like Weight Watchers which takes a sensible and healthful approach to losing weight. Be wary of diet organizations that are costly or limit you to their own foods.
- Be patient. More permanent results will be obtained if weight loss is gradual. Remember that it takes time for the body to adjust to its new programmng.
- Some studies indicate that when there is an inadequate intake of essential nutrients, fat is not burned efficiently which may contribute to obesity.
- Sugar in the form of soda pop, candy, cookies, cake, ice cream and pastries is responsible for much of childhood obesity. Salted snack foods such as potato chips and corn chips are as much as 40 percent fat. Many breakfast cereals are up to 60 percent sugar. Making these foods unavailable to family members can go a long way in the fight against obesity.
- Emphasize the following foods: Lentils, beans, plain baked potatoes, baked squash, brown rice, whole grain breads (low fat or no fat), white fish, white chicken, skim milk, low-fat cottage cheese, no-fat yogurt, turkey, fresh fruits and vegetables. Restrict your intake of avocados, figs, bananas, white rice, sweet potatoes, coconut and corn.

- Avoid high-fat dairy products like cheese, sour cream, ice cream, butter, whole milk, and rich dressings. Eliminate soda pop, mayonnaise, fried foods, red meats, gravies, custards, pastries, cakes, peanut butter and junk foods from your diet.
- Do not eat too little. Any diet that is less than 1200 calories is critical for the maintenance of good health and the promotion of permanent weight loss. In addition, all diets should contain some percentage of desirable fat which can be ingested in the form of olive or safflower oil. Supplementing your diet with one or two teaspoons of these oils is thought to actually improve the burning of fat.
- Use digestive enzymes before every meal.
- Do not consume alcohol—all alcoholic beverages are high in calories.
- Fiber supplements can be taken in the form of guar gum or glucomannan.
- Avoid artificial sweeteners. There is some evidence that artificial sweeteners can actually increase appetite and result in weight gain.
- Barley malt sweetener can be used instead of sugar.
- Omit all substances which are thought to be appetite stimulants. Some of the most common are salt, hot spices, coffee, tea, tobacco and sugar.
- Avoid any fad diets that are designed around a high-protein, low-carbohydrate diet. This combination, if eaten over a long period of time, poses some significant health hazards.
- Weigh yourself regularly and record your weight on a chart. If you go up three pounds from your ideal weight, adjust your diet and exercise to lose those three pounds. It is so much easier to lose three pounds than to lose twenty.
- Stay off the diet roller coaster of overeating and then crash dieting. Keep a consistently healthy lifestyle centered around sensible eating and regular exercise.
- Keep your kitchen stocked with healthy low-fat/low-sugar snacks.

REFLECTIONS ON WEIGHT LOSS STRATEGIES

Unquestionably, short term weight loss programs fail to completely address the total biochemical processes involved in not only burning fat stores, but also in preventing future fat storage. So many people are concerned about their expanding waistlines, it's no wonder they reach for quick-fix diet plans that usually ignore the long term effects of radical weight loss strategies. Liquid diets, diets high in protein, diets that promote bizarre foods and diets that disrupt the normal pH balance of the body are only some of the typical drastic weight loss programs currently in use. Clearly, most weight-loss plans stress the physical body. In so doing, they at best, provide only a temporary solution to the problem.

Ideally, a sensible weight loss program should employ a nutritional strategy which works in tandem with body systems to maximize fat burning capabilities. Successful weight management depends on fully understanding human biochemistry, and in so doing targeting those physiological processes which expedite weight reduction. When given the proper tools, the human body has an inherent ability to effectively manage its weight. The key to boosting this ability lies in creating a biological equilibrium between all body systems by integrating nutrition, exercise and the proper supplementation.

A SUMMARY OF WHAT TO LOOK FOR IN WEIGHT-LOSS PRODUCTS

Fiber Supplements

Psyllium-based products are the most common type of fiber supplements. Italian studies have found that in a reducing diet for women who averaged about 60 percent overweight, weight loss was greater when plantain or psyllium was added to the diet. It appears that psyllium produced weight loss by limiting caloric intake die to it appetite-satiating effect and by reducing the intestinal absorption of lipids. Good formulas combine different types of fibers and often add various herbs such as guar gum to tone the colon and promote better elimination and digestion.

Liquid Protein Supplements

Several protein-replacement powders and liquids exist which can help facilitate the creation of lean muscle mass and the burning of fat. Spirulina-based and soy-based products are an excellent source of usable proteins and when other nutrients, fat emulsifiers and dietary aids are added to formulas, these products can serve as good meal replacements. Good supplements include a complete array of amino acids, enzymes, antioxidants and an assortment of vitamins, minerals and specific herbs which facilitate weight loss and promote regularity.

Fat-Burning Formulas

The most effective fat-burning combinations include 1) the herb ephedra, 2) a natural caffeine-containing plant such as kola nut or guarana and 3) some source of salicylic acid such as white willow or aspirin. Adding *Garcinia cambogia* (citrin), chromium picolinate, chitosan or amino acids such as carnitine or methionine can further potentiate the mix. Taking ephedra alone is not recommended as dosages must be too high to be effective. Any thermogenic formula designed to burn calories off as heat can create some unpleasant side effects and should not be used by pregnant or nursing women, nor by anyone suffering from hypertension, heart disease, adrenal or thyroid disorders or anxiety attacks.

Natural Appetite Suppressants

The best natural appetite suppressants include phenylalanine and tyrosine combined with *Garcinia cambogia* (citrin) or glucomannan. Other ingredients such as herbs which discourage eating and minerals such as manganese or potassium citrate help to make the formula even more effective. Chromium picolinate is also used in supplements designed to fight food cravings, stabilize blood sugar, and promote the creation of lean muscle mass.

CONCLUSION

Typically, most weight loss programs expect the body to respond to a drastic alteration of diet and activity with no prior physiological preparation. Being overweight is frequently treated as a disease. Consequently, the *symptoms* of obesity are targeted rather than addressing and correcting the *cause* of obesity.

The purpose of this book has been to offer the reader natural alternatives which work to suppress the appetite and enhance the burning of fat. The best phen-fen alternatives appear to be the amino acids discussed which raise brain serotonin and dopamine levels. These amino acids can be used in conjunction with a variety of other natural compounds which suppress the appetite, encourage the formation of lean muscle mass, help stabilize blood sugar, promote the burning of fat, stimulate better bowel and kidney function, and support the thyroid, liver and the adrenal glands.

Looking for various products that satisfy these parameters is encouraged. In addition, a number of separate supplements can be purchased which serve to support each other synergistically and create effective and permanent weight loss.

The exercise factor has not been discussed at length in this book but exercise would naturally boost any weight loss strategy. The notion that only powerful, expensive and potentially dangerous drugs can suppress the appetite and create successful weight loss is simply not true. For every synthetic or pharmaceutical drug, an alternative compound exists in nature. Consider the following list:

APPETITE SUPPRESSANTS:
Phen-fen   vs.   phenylalanine, tyrosine and methionine

FAT BINDERS:
Orlistat   vs.   chitosan

FAT BURNERS:
Leptin or Sibutramine vs.   ephedra, caffeine, salicylic acid

As more attention is focused on safer, more natural substances, weight-loss formulas will continue to improve. The role of hormones like DHEA and melatonin are only now beginning to surface and their therapeutic implications could be profound. If you feel like pharmaceutical agents such as phen-fen are your only hope, think again. Mother Nature has provided a vast array of safe and effective compounds which can significantly contribute to healthy and permanent weight loss.

ENDNOTES

1. L. Chaitow, "Amino Acids in Therapy." (Thorsons, 1985) and "Slimming and Health Workbook." (Thorsons, 1989).
2. G. Enzi et al., "Effect of a hydrophilic mucilage in the treatment of obese patients," *Pharmatherapeutica*, 2 (7): 1980, 412-28.
3. Jon J. Michnovicz. *How to Reduce Your Risk of Breast Cancer*. (New York: Warner Book Inc. 1994) 54.
4. T.B. Van Tallie. Obesity: adverse effects on health and longevity. *American Journal of Clinical Nutrition*. (1979) 32: L Suppl: 2723-33.
5. Elizabeth Somer, M.A., R.D., *Nutrition for Women*. (New York: Henry Holt and Company, 1993), 273.
6. Ibid., 274.
7. Ibid., 281.
8. J. L. Nauss, J.L. Thompson and J. Nagyvary. *The binding of micellar lipids to chitosan*. Department of Biochemistry and Biophysiology, Texas A&M University 1983, 18(10), 714-19.
9. J. Abelin and A. Lassus. "Fat binder as a weight reducer in patients with moderate obesity." *ARS Medicina*, (Helsinki, Aug-October, 1994).
10. Yuji Maezaki, Keisuke Tsuji et al., "Hypocholesterolemic effect of chitosan in adult males." *Biosci-C\Biotchnol-Biochem*, 1993: 57(9) 1439-44.
11. Takaaki Kobayashi et al., "Effect of chitosan on serum and liver cholesterol levels in cholesterol-fed rats," *Nutritional Rep. Int.*, 1979: 19(3), 327-34.
12. Michihiro Sugano, et al., "Hypocholesterolemic effects of chitosan in cholesterol-fed rats," *Nutritional Rep. Int.* 1978: 18(5) 531-7.
13. George Vahouny, et al., "Comparative effects of chitosan and cholestryramine on lymphatic absorption of lipids in the rat," School of Medical Health Science, *American Journal of Clinical Nutrition*, 1983: 38(2) 278-84.
14. Shiegeo Suzuki, et al., "Chitin and chitosan oligomers as hypolipemics and formulations containing them," *Jpn. Kokai Tokkyo Koho JP*, Feb. 22 1988, Appl. 86/184662.
15. Ikuo Ikeda, et al., "Interrelated effects of dietary fiber and fat as lymphatic cholesterol and triglyceride absorption in rats," *Journal of Nutrition*, 1989: 119(10) 1383-7.
16. J.G. LeHoux and F. Grondin, "Some effects of chitosan on liver function in the rat," *Endocrinology*. 1993: March 132(3): 1078-84.
17. Hideo Kato, et al., "Chitosan as antihypertensive," *Jpn. Kikoi Tokkyo Koho JP*, 01 March 1994, appl. 92/147759.
18. Hideo Kato, et al., "Mechanism of the rise in blood pressure by sodium chloride and decrease effect of chitosan on blood pressure," *Baiosaiensu to Indasutori*, 1993 51(12), 987-8.
19. Satoshi Nakamura, et al., "Chitosan for enhancement of bioavailability of calcium," *Jpn. Kokai Tokkyo Koho JP*, Aug, 1995, appl. 93/355022.

20. Fujiio Ito, et al., "Role of chitosan as a supplementary food for osteoporosis," *Gekkan Fudo Kemikaru*, 1995, 11(2), 39-44.

21. Osamu Kanauchi, et al., "Mechanism for the inhibition of fat digestion by chitosan and for the synergistic effect of ascorbate," *Biosci-Biotech-Biochem.*, 1995, 59(5), 786-90.

22. A.A. Conte, "A non-prescription alternative in weight reduction therapy," *The Bariatrician Summer.* 1993, 17-19.

23. *American Journal of Clinical Nutrition*, 1977.

24. Muhammed Majeed, Ph.D., *Citric: A Revolutionary Herbal Approach to Weight Management*, 1994.

25. Ann Louise Gittleman, M.S. *Super Nutrition for Women* and D. Ricquier et al., "An immunological study of the uncoupling protein of brown adipose tissue mitochondria," *Biochem Jour*, 1983, 210, 859-66.

26. Brain K. Bailey D.P.M. and Susan Smith Jones, Ph.D. "Ten ways to increase your metabolism," *Let's Live*, August, 1994.

27. G. Bush and D. Bush, *New England Journal of Medicine*, 1986, 315, 1519-24, W.D. Drucker et l., "Biologic activity of dehydroepiandrosterone sulfate (DHEA) in man," *Journal of Clinical Endocrinology*, 35, 1972, 48-54.

28. DHEA Replacement Therapy, Life Extension Report, September, 1993, vol. 13, (9), 66.

29. C. Branco-Castelo et al., "Circulating hormone levels in menopausal women receiving different hormone replacement therapy regiments: A comparison." *Journal-Repro-Med*, August, 1995, 40 (8), 556-60.

30. J.R. Porter, et al., "The effects of discontinuing dehydroepiandrosterone supplementation on Zucker rat food intake and hypothalamic neurotransmitter," *Int-Jour-Obes-Relate-Metab-Disorders*, July, 1995: 19 (7), 480-88.

31. R. Sciborski, "The influence of DHEA on serum lipids, insulin and sex hormone levels in rabbits with induced hypercholesterolemia," *Gynecol-Endocrinol*, March, 1995: 9 (1), 23-28.

32. G. DePergola et al., "Low dehydroepiandrosterone circulating levels in premenopausal obese women with very high body mass index," *Metabolism*, February, 1991: 40(2), 187-90.

33. "DHEA Replacement Therapy," *Life Extension Report*, 66.

34. Ibid.

35. R.T. Stanko, et al., "Body composition, energy utilization and nitrogen metabolism with a 4.25-MJ/d low energy diet supplemented with pyruvate," *American Journal of Clinical Nutrition*, 1992, 56, 630-35.

36. Ibid.

37. Emile G. Bliznakov, M.D. and Gerald L. Hunt. *The Miracle Nutrient: Coenzyme Q10.* (New York: Bantam Books, 1989), 153.

38. Shelley Beattie and John Romano, "The Ten Best Performance Supplements," *Muscular Development and Fitness*, July, 1995, 50, 192.

39. L. Bukowiecki, et al., "Ephedrine, a potential slimming drug, directly stimulates thermogenesis in brown adipocytes via B-adrenoreceptors," *Inter Jour Obes*, 1982, (6), 343-50. L. Landsberg, et al., "Sympathoadrenal activity and obesity: physiological rational for the use

of adrenergic thermogenic drugs," *Inter Jour Obes*, 1993, (17) suppl 1, s29-34.

40. See A. Astrup et al., "Enhanced thermogenic responsiveness during chronic ephedrine treatment in man." *Am Jour Clin Nutri*, 1985, (42), 83-94 and R.S. Schawarts et al., " Reduced thermogenic effect of feeding in obesity: role of norepinephrine," *Metabolism*, 1983, (32), 114-17.

41. T. Yoshida et al., "Thermogenic, antiobesity effects of bofutsusho-san in MSG-obese mice," *Inter Jour Obes*, 1993, (17, suppl 1, S35-40.

42. *Journal of Clinical Pharmacology*, 1975, (9), 193-98.

43. A.G. Dulloo and D.S. Miller, "Reversal of obesity in the genetically obese fa/fa Zucker rat with an ephedrine/methylxanthines thermogenic mixture," *Jour Nutri*, 1987, (117), 383-89. See also A. G. Dulloo and D.S. Miller, "The thermogenic properties of ephedrin/methyl xanthine mixtures: animal studies," *Am Jour Clin Nutri*, 1986, (43), 388-94.

44. A.G. Dulloo et al., "Potentiation of the thermogenic antiobesity effects of ephedrine by dietary methylxanthines: Adenosine antagonism or phosphodiesterase inhibition?" *Metabolism*, 1992, 41 (11), 1233-41. A. Astrup et al., "Thermogenic synergism between ephedrine and caffeine in healthy volunteers, a double-blind placebo-controlled study," *Metabolism*, 1991, 40, 323-29. A. Astrup et al., "Pharmacology of thermogenic drugs," *Amer Jour Clini Nutri*, 1992, 550246S-8S. A. G. Dulloo, "Ephedrine, xanthines and prostaglandin-inhibitors: actions and interactions in the stimulation of thermogenesis," *Int Jour Obes*, 1993, 17, suppl 1, S35-40.

45. T.J. Horton and C.A. Geissler, "Aspirin potentiates the effect of ephedrine on the thermogenic response to a meal in obese but not lean women," *Int Jour Obes*, 1991, 15, 359-66.

46. A.G. Dulloo and D.S. Miller, "The thermogenic properties of ephedrine/methyl xanthine mixtures: animal studies," *Am Jour Clin Nutri*, 1986, 43, 388-94.

47. Ibid.

48. Ibid.

49. J. Groen, et al., "Extracts of glycyrrhizinic acid on the electrolyte metabolism in Addison's disease," *Jour of Clini Investi*, 1952, 31, 87-91.

50. Daniel B. Mowrey, Ph.D., *The Scientific Validation of Herbal Medicine*, (Keats Publishing, New Canaan, Connecticut: 1986), 26.

51. R. Wurtman, "Aspartase effects on brain serotonin," *American Journal of Clinical Nutrition*, 1987, 45: 799-801. See also R. Wurtman, "Neurochemical changes following high-dose aspartase with dietary carbohydrates," *New England Journal of Medicine*, 1983, 389: 429-30 and R. Wurtman, "Possible effect on seizure susceptibility," *Lancet*, 1985, 2: 1060.

52. John Olney, *The Journal of Neuropathology and Experimental Neurology*, 1996.

53. Linda Linda, Bill Bonvie and Donna Gates, *The Stevia Story*. (B.E.D., Atlanta, Georgia: 1997), 53.

54. Ibid., 38.

55. Ibid.

56. Richard Passwater Ph.D. *GTF Chromium.* (New Canaan, Connecticut: Keats Publishing, 1982), 11.
57. D.E. Walsh, et al., "Effect of glucomannan on obese patients: A clinical study," *Int Jour Obes,* 1984, 8 (4): 289-93.
58. Betty Kamen, "Gymnema Extract," *Let's Live,* Sept. 1989, 40-41.
59. *Journal of Ethnopharmacology,* 1986, 143-46.
60. R. Passwater, "Glutamine, the Surprising Brain Fuel," Educational pamphlet. See also R.Williams, *Nutrition Against Disease,* (Bantam Books, 1981).
61. Michael T. Murray, N.D., *The Healing Power of Herbs,* (Prima Publishing, Rocklin, California: 1995), 123.
62. Richard Pardee, *Muscle and Fitness,* September, 1985.
63. D.H. Dean and R.N. Hiramoto, "Weight loss during pancreatin feeding of rats," *Nutrition Reports International,* 1984, 29: 167-72.
64. J.W. Anderson and C.A. Bryant,"Dietary Fiber, Diabetes and Obesity," *Am. J. Gastroenterol.,* 1986, 898-906.
65. Ohnishi F. Nomura and Y Satomura, *Int. J. Obesity,* 1986,
66. G.J. Naylor, et al., "A double-blind placebo controlled trial of ascorbic acid in obesity," *Nutr Health,* 1985, 4:25-28. And G.J. Naylor, "A double-blind placebo controlled trial of ascorbic acid in obesity," *IRCS Med Sci,* 1982, 10: 848.